Live Free from
ASTHMA and ALLERGIES

Live Free from
ASTHMA and ALLERGIES

Use the BioSET System to Detoxify and Desensitize Your Body

REVISED

ELLEN W. CUTLER, DC

CELESTIAL ARTS
Berkeley | Toronto

CA

Celestial Arts
an imprint of Ten Speed Press
PO Box 7123
Berkeley, California 94707

Distributed in Australia by Simon and Schuster Australia, in Canada by Ten Speed Press Canada, in New Zealand by Southern Publishers Group, in South Africa by Real Books, and in the United Kingdom and Europe by Publishers Group UK.

Cover design by: Katy Brown
Text design by: Jeff Brandenburg

Material on p. 134 reprinted with permission from *The Energy Within* by Richard M. Chin. Copyright © 1995 by Richard M. Chin, Marlowe & Company, New York, NY.

ISBN-13: 978-1-58761-301-2

Printed in the United States of America
Originally published as *Winning the War Against Asthma and Allergies*, 1998.

Contents

PART ONE | Sensitivities: Types, Causes, Symptoms, Testing, and Treatments

PART TWO | Asthma: Warning Signs, Symptoms, Respiratory Diseases, Causes, and Preventive Measures

PART THREE | BioSET (Bioenergetic Sensitivity and Enzyme Therapy)

PART FOUR | Adjunctive Therapy

PART FIVE | Case Studies

Appendices

This book is dedicated to all the asthmatics and allergic people who read it, benefit from it, and put it to use to clear their sensitivities and regain their health and vitality.

Acknowledgments

I would like to thank many people who supported me and contributed to the completion of this book's revision.

My special thanks and gratitude go to Jo Ann Deck for having the fortitude to take on this revision of *Live Free from Asthma and Allergies*. Surely without her support and determination, this book would not have been published. I would like to especially thank my editor, Joy Parker. She is perfect—I can't really say much more. She has my deep-felt appreciation for outstanding work. Again, she is perfect. I would also like to thank Eve Cantwell who came in at the last minute for some touch-up and refining. I would also like to thank my editor at Celestial Arts, Lisa Westmoreland, who is not only bright and talented but absolutely a joy to work with. I would also like to thank the staff at the BioSET clinic.

And special thanks to the BioSET practitioners who undertook the task of research for the in-depth information presented in the appendix: Mauree Kai; Elissa Blesch, LAc; Darshan Khalsa, LAc; Bernie Epstein, DC, LAc, CCN, DACBN; and Nelson Bulmash, DC, ND, CCN, DACBN.

I would also like to acknowledge my most precious children, Aaron and Gabrielle. They are the light in my life.

And I cannot forget Claire Pogue, who made possible the first edition of this asthma book. She will always be remembered and I will always be grateful.

Foreword

There is a light at the end of the tunnel for those who suffer from allergies and asthma. Much of it is contained in Ellen Cutler's new book, *Live Free from Asthma and Allergies*.

As a board-certified physician in pediatric and adult allergy and immunology, I was initially very skeptical of all forms of complementary medicine. However, after developing chronic sinus infections and food allergies fifteen or sixteen years ago, I soon found that Western medicine did not have all the answers. After years of antibiotics, antihistamines, nasal steroids, decongestants, mucous thinners, and elimination diets, I was sicker than before. Chronic fatigue, body aches, headaches, and nausea were my daily companions. I saw every specialist in allopathic medicine and was basically told that I would have to live with my symptoms.

With nowhere to go, one of my patients suggested I see her family herbalist, who had successfully treated her many times. Reluctantly, I found my way to his office. With a combination of three herbs and two vitamins, I felt great within one week. This herbal practitioner and his five herbs had beaten the best allopathic physicians I knew. My curiosity peaked and I had to learn more.

A friend of mine dared me to take an acupuncture course for physicians, and for the next two years I studied its effect on pain, allergies, and asthma in my practice. I did see much improvement in many of my patients and myself, but there was something missing. I still had some food allergies.

At that point I was given Dr. Cutler's book, *The Food Allergy Cure*. After a few conversations with several of my colleagues, I learned that this doctor was someone who had a slightly different approach.

I attended one of Dr. Cutler's seminars and was very impressed with her knowledge of enzymes, allergies, and Western medicine. Her approach (called BioSET) combined treatment with enzymes for digestion and systemic therapy, homeopathic remedies for detoxification, and a very innovative natural allergy desensitization protocol. That was the magic combination for me and many of my patients. You must detoxify and cleanse the body, as well as optimize digestion and eliminate allergies, to achieve the best results in successfully treating asthma.

I had been studying the BioSET method for roughly one year when I received a call from Dr. Cutler's office. She had decided to add an MD degree to her already long list of achievements. Part of her training included proctorships where she would spend two-week rotations with Western medical doctors in various sub-specialties. She wanted to know whether I would allow her to spend two weeks with me at my office, seeing patients from a Western medicine perspective. I said to myself, "Let's see . . . two weeks of one-on-one with Ellen Cutler or two weeks by myself?" I made that decision in a heartbeat!

Ellen came to Redlands, California, and for two weeks we saw all of my patients together. I have to tell you that this was one of the greatest learning experiences of my life. This is when I really learned BioSET. With her added input, many of my most difficult patients were evaluated and treated, and they markedly improved. For example, I have one patient who suffered from stubborn chronic sinus infections—several years later, he is still on the same two natural products that Ellen recommended and rarely has sinus infections anymore.

During the past few years since my one-on-one with Ellen, her BioSET principles have allowed me to treat some of my worst patients, whose illnesses include steroid-dependent asthma, steroid-dependent eczema, fibromyalgia, chronic sinusitis, and urticaria.

If you are a layperson who suffers from allergies or immune conditions, this book will explain your illness and how to treat it from A to Z, utilizing both Western and BioSET methods of treatment. If you are a health care practitioner and have not yet discovered BioSET, you need to read *Live Free from Asthma and Allergies* and incorporate its principles into your practice. The rewards will be well worth the effort.

—*Jim Munsen*

Introduction

All over the world, BioSET (Bioenergetic Sensitivity and Enzyme Therapy) practitioners are treating patients of all ages who want to conquer their asthma and their food and environmental sensitivities. Not only do these patients reduce or often overcome their need to use asthma medication through BioSET, but many of them say farewell to the disease permanently. The victory is sweet indeed.

"As an acute asthma sufferer," wrote one patient, "I've had to fight daily battles, using medication and avoidance to foods and substances that cause me to react. But with BioSET I've been able to win not only the battles, but the war forever." The road to complete recovery is short and easy for some patients, long and arduous for others, but it is a journey that is well worth every challenge.

About twenty million Americans suffer from asthma, 6.9 million of them children.[1] In the last twenty years, despite advances in medical treatment and medication, the incidence of asthma among women and children and the number of fatalities caused by asthma have more than doubled. When I hear these statistics, I want to shout, "There is an answer! There is a way to conquer asthma!" This book is my declaration to everyone who struggles with asthma that there is a complementary therapy that can defeat this life-threatening disease.

My work with food and environmental sensitivities started almost twenty years ago and eventually led me to write this book. In my clinical experience with all types of chronically ill individuals, three contributing factors have repeatedly presented themselves: toxicity, poor digestion and dietary stress, and sensitivities. Although this book focuses on the relationship between sensitivities and asthma, it can benefit all those who suffer from sensitivities or any other chronic health problems.

Many asthmatics live with symptoms every day of their lives. They experience heaviness in their chest, breathing difficulties, and perhaps some coughing or wheezing. They often find themselves struggling for oxygen, a problem that normal individuals rarely think about. Asthmatics may develop these symptoms in response to foods, molds, chemicals, or a variety of other substances, as well as to changes in temperature, humidity, or other environmental factors. These reactions can happen in seconds, and they can be life threatening, as I have repeatedly witnessed at my clinic over twenty-five years.

There is little doubt that asthma is exacerbated by sensitivities (allergies). Asthmatics are affected by many sensitivities, ranging from sensitivities to chemicals, such as formaldehyde in perfumes; new clothing, carpets, and plastics; chlorine and fluoride in the water supply; hydrocarbons in car exhaust; and trichloroethylene in dry-cleaned garments, to sensitivities to natural substances, such as textiles, pollens, milk, feathers, yeast and fungus, viruses, and bacteria, and even to sensitivities to stressful and negative emotions.

How This Book Is Structured

This book is divided into six main sections: sensitivities, asthma, BioSET, adjunctive therapy, cases studies, and appendices. Chapter 14 offers case histories documenting the results of BioSET. I suggest that you read it first, even before chapter 1; it will help you truly appreciate why the information in this book is a must-read for all those who suffer from asthma and food and environmental sensitivities.

Part 1 discusses sensitivities. Chapters one through three explain the types, origins, and causes of sensitivities and summarize the various sensitivity testing and treatment approaches, including BioSET. This section defines the expanded meaning of "allergies," which I prefer to refer to as "sensitivities."

Part 2 presents a discussion on asthma. Chapters 4 through 7 review the symptoms of asthma and the numerous sensitivities that can trigger an asthma sufferer. These sensitivities include food, hormones, glands, vitamins, funguses, viruses, bacteria, cold, humidity, mold, pollen, dust, animals, salicylates (analgesics), chemicals, metabolic imbalances, and genetic factors. Anything can be a potential sensitivity, even medications such as aspirin and birth control pills. Once a BioSET practitioner identifies an individual's sensitivities, their cause can be eliminated and they may no longer pose a problem.

Chapter 8 is a complete guide to creating a sensitivity-free environment for asthma sufferers. Once people have completed their BioSET clearings, many of these suggestions no longer need be followed. But until a person's sensitivities are eliminated, this chapter can be extremely helpful to all who suffer from them, especially asthmatics.

Part 3 outlines the uses of BioSET. Chapters 9, 10, and 11 delineate the most common treatment and clearing protocols—including clearing the home and clearing the self during an emergency—for the many different types of asthmatics, including children and infants. These three chapters describe in detail the revolutionary aspects of BioSET therapy, which has so transformed the lives of many asthmatics. For instance, imagine for a moment that your son or daughter could be triggered, without warning, into a life-threatening asthma attack that left them unable to breathe or even call out for help. Childhood asthma can be a living nightmare for parents. Yet every day, BioSET practitioners see children who suffer from chronic asthma symptoms undergo complementary therapies that eventually transform them into normal, healthy, asthma-free kids. As they watch their own lives and the lives of their children completely turn around, these parents often ask me why BioSET is not the mainstream approach to treating sensitivities and asthma.

Chapter 12 reveals ways to increase the energy levels and stamina of those with sensitivities, further enhancing quality of life.

An Overview of Enzyme Therapy

In addition to breathing problems, most asthmatics appear to suffer from poor digestion, including constipation, diarrhea, bloating, and irritable bowel syndrome. Many are carbohydrate intolerant, unable to sufficiently digest and utilize the nutrients in sugars and carbohydrates of all types. In essence, they are deficient in critical, life-supporting enzymes that are needed for every chemical reaction in our bodies. These enzymes work to build our bodies from proteins, fats, and carbohydrates. No vitamin or mineral can function without enzyme support. Of the more than five thousand enzymes that have been discovered, four are food enzymes found in raw food, twenty-two are digestive enzymes made by the pancreas, and the rest are metabolic enzymes, which involve all the body's different systems and help maintain a healthy immune system.

I learned about enzymes from Edward Howell, MD, one of the foremost pioneers in enzyme therapy. His research initiated an exciting new phase in the study of nutrition and its implications for asthma and other chronic health problems. According to Dr. Howell, all asthmatics suffer enzyme deficiency as a result of poor digestion, which eventually compromises immune system function.

Part 4 introduces enzyme therapy as an adjunctive therapy. Chapter 13 is a complete overview of enzyme therapy, including how it is used, why it is important for asthmatics, and why proper digestion and utilization of foods is paramount to health and vitality.

Part 5, as mentioned above, shares case histories. And part 6 includes three appendices. Appendix A covers specific foods related to dietary stress, and food and materials containing key allergens. Appendix B contains miscellaneous resources, filters, allergen-free products, and foods. Appendix C contains new research on asthma. There is also an endnotes section, a glossary, and a bibliography.

Life Free from Asthma

The information provided in this book can help you reduce your risk of death from asthma by helping you to identify and eliminate its true causes. It can enable you to see yourself not as an asthmatic, but as an individual with your own unique biochemical makeup, sensitivities, and needs. Most asthmatics have been told that asthma is a chronic problem they will have to contend with for the rest of their lives. This book shows that asthma can be defeated, not miraculously and instantaneously, but gradually and permanently, once the sensitivities that cause it have been eliminated, your diet restructured, your digestion restored, and your body rid of as many toxins as possible.

Every asthmatic should be able to lead a normal life. If you're an asthma sufferer who wants to take control of your condition or your children's asthma, then read this book to discover how you can secure optimal health and conquer this disease. I encourage you to tell others about this book and BioSET and then form support groups where you can share information, test each other, and even clear sensitivities. BioSET Institute would be willing to help with support and provide answers to any questions you may have. Refer to our website, www.bioset.net, for more information on support and guidance. If you're a health practitioner dealing with the asthma and sensitivities of your patients and/or loved ones, this book will introduce you to a new approach that may revolutionize your practice. Check out the website for courses in your area and online. You may even wish to become a BioSET practitioner yourself.

In the twenty-first century, the growing incidence of asthma reflects three factors:

+ An increase of chemical pollutants in our environment and our food

+ An exponential rise in the use of pharmaceutical drugs that may, over time, weaken and suppress the immune system

+ A decline in adequate nutrition, caused in large measure by poor absorption of vitamins, minerals, and other nutrients, due in part to eating too quickly or "on the go" and not chewing well enough

Fortunately, the twenty-first century also heralds a new awakening to drug-free complementary approaches to chronic health problems. People are disillusioned with the conventional establishment and are demanding remedies that enliven their bodies and minds and encourage, rather than suppress, their own innate healing force. We all need a chance to reclaim control of and responsibility for our health. This book offers an empowering new understanding of the symptoms and causes of asthma and a complementary approach to overcoming it—now and forever.

PART ONE

Sensitivities: Types, Causes, Symptoms, Testing, and Treatments

Defining Sensitivities

In this book we will be exploring the relationship between allergies or, as I prefer to call them, "sensitivities," and asthma. A sensitivity, as I use the term in this book, is the body's abnormal, adverse physical reaction to certain substances, commonly known as allergens (or antigens). While these substances can be either toxic, such as exhaust fumes or other petrochemicals, or nontoxic, such as pollens or food, those who suffer from sensitivities will react to them in quantities that are harmless to most people.

Developing a Sensitivity: Allergens and Antibodies

When exposed to allergens, sensitive individuals develop an excess of an antibody called immunoglobulin E (IgE). The IgE antibodies react with allergens to release histamines and other chemicals from cell tissues, producing various sensitivity symptoms. In other words, the immune system mistakenly identifies harmless substances as dangerous invaders and activates an antibody attack to defend the body. The development of an allergy begins with sensitization to the substance on first contact, usually without symptoms. Only upon reexposure do the previously created antibodies become active and produce symptoms.

COMMON SENSITIVITIES AND
THE TEN BASIC SENSITIVITIES

Although a person can develop allergies to practically any substance, the most common allergens include pollen, dust, dust mites, animal dander (skin, saliva, hair, or fur), feathers, cosmetics, mold, insect venom, certain chemicals, drugs, medicines (especially penicillin), and foods. The most troublesome foods are usually peanuts, other tree nuts, shellfish, milk, egg, wheat, and soy. Allergens may cause a reaction following inhalation, injection, ingestion, or contact with the skin. While sensitivity reactions can involve any part of the body, they most frequently affect the nose, chest, skin, and eyes. The rarest and most dangerous type of reaction, called anaphylactic shock, can affect many organs at once, causing a rapid decrease in blood pressure, a rash or hives, breathing difficulties, abdominal pain, a swollen tongue or throat, diarrhea, fainting, asphyxiation, and, all too often, death.

There are ten basic sensitivities:

+ Amino acids
+ Biochemicals
+ Fatty acids
+ Minerals
+ Phenolics
+ Sugars
+ Vitamin A
+ B vitamins
+ Vitamin C
+ Vitamin E

A BROAD DEFINITION OF SENSITIVITIES

Between thirty-five and fifty million people in the United States suffer from some type of significant allergy.[1] These types of reactions can emerge suddenly at any age without prior warning. Many studies have shown conclusively that parents with sensitivities will tend to have children with sensitivities. However, research suggests that what is inherited is simply the tendency to develop a sensitivity of *some kind*, not of any particular type. Regardless, in my practice I have repeatedly seen that a child's allergic tendencies are often related to his or her parents' sensitivities, and I have often treated parents and their children for the same kinds of sensitivities. Certain people (known as "atopic") tend to be more susceptible to these types of reactions, and once these individuals develop one sensitivity, others commonly follow.

Part of the difficulty in determining the exact number of allergy sufferers lies in how broadly or narrowly one defines the term. Medical doctors and scientists often maintain a narrow definition, asserting that the only *true* allergies are those that result from the activation of IgE antibodies. However, millions of people experience symptoms of sensitivity to a food or substance without the antibody reaction. These people can be said to have an intolerance or a hypersensitivity to particular substances. Although the causes may differ, the diagnosis and treatment of sensitivities and intolerances often overlap. As a result, allergy research and information benefits more kinds of people than just those with traditional allergies.

In my clinical work I have found that the measurements and treatments used for many allergies, sensitivities, and intolerances are exactly the same. Therefore, in my practice I use the terms interchangeably. (As mentioned, for this book I will use the term "sensitivity" instead of allergy.)

Sensitivities can also cause a predisposition to colds and flus by compromising the immune system and lowering the body's resistance. Once the body becomes host to viruses and bacteria, it can be difficult to distinguish a cold from an allergic reaction, especially since they often occur simultaneously. However, sensitivities don't generally cause fever, and colds should not linger for more than a week or two, unlike sensitivities, which may refuse to go away.

Taking the wider view of a sensitivity as any negative or abnormal response in the immune system, I believe there is no such thing as a simple cold. A cold is the response of a challenged immune system, whether it be responding to a food, a pollen, or a virus. Since a virus can also be considered an allergen, I treat a cold like a sensitivity, with excellent results.

Causes and Origins of Sensitivities

A sensitivity reaction can be IgE mediated or non-IgE mediated. An IgE-mediated sensitivity is the traditional type, recognized by most medical doctors, in which immunoglobulin E antibodies are produced in response to environmental allergens and foods. Typical symptoms are hay fever and some forms of eczema. A non-IgE-mediated allergy, which conventional physicians do not always recognize as a sensitivity, is a negative change in the immune system that can cause a variety of symptoms, such as a headache or irritability. Allergens or sensitivities that are non-IgE mediated may also affect the sympathetic and parasympathetic nervous systems. For example, in the case of asthma, when the lungs are irritated by sensitivities to dust, smoke, perfume, or bacteria, the parasympathetic nervous system may be stimulated to secrete acetylcholine. When this happens, acetylcholine constricts bronchial muscles and increases mucus production, thereby triggering an asthmatic attack.

Allergens or sensitivities such as bacteria, viruses, or certain foods seem to create antigen-antibody complexes by combining with the T and B cells, the body's adaptive defense system produced in the bone marrow. These antigen-antibody complexes lodge themselves in certain tissues, for example, in the lungs or bronchioles of asthmatics. In an attempt to destroy these complexes, the immune system produces an autoimmune reaction that inflames and destroys healthy tissue. This inflammation triggers an asthma attack and creates a chronic condition until the sensitivities and complexes are removed.

GENETIC OR INHERITED ALLERGIES

The most common cause of allergies is genetic. The probability of developing a sensitivity is increased if one or both parents suffer from any type of allergic condition. In fact, this factor is the strongest when predicting allergies in offspring. When one parent has allergies, the child will develop allergies 75 percent of the time. If both parents have allergies, the child will develop sensitivities 100 percent of the time.

In addition, when an expectant mother is exposed to various toxins, such as chemicals or radiation, or even suffers an illness, such as a flu or infection, allergies and/or sensitivities will often develop in her unborn child. Altered cells do not carry over the original genetic codes and do not undergo normal development. As a result, the child's organs and tissues may develop nonfunctional sensory nerve receptors that are unable to conduct messages to and from the spinal cord and brain. In some children these nerve receptors become hyposensitive toward certain items, in others they become hypersensitive. When hyposensitive fibers predominate, we may see not only a few sensitivity reactions, but also poor growth, chronic fatigue, and poor functioning of body and mind.

POOR DIGESTION

The second most common cause of sensitivities is poor digestion. If a food is not properly digested, it will eventually trigger a sensitivity reaction in the body.

One common result of poor digestion is leaky gut syndrome, a common medical condition in which the intestinal lining is more porous than usual. These large openings between the cells of the intestinal wall allow toxic materials that would normally be eliminated from the body to pass into the bloodstream. The primary cause of leaky gut syndrome is inflammation of the intestinal lining, usually brought on by one or more of the following factors:

+ Antibiotics, which allow the overgrowth of harmful bacteria in the gastrointestinal tract

- Foods and beverages that are contaminated by parasites
- Deficiencies of digestive enzymes such as lactase, which breaks down lactose (milk sugar)
- Nonsteroidal anti-inflammatory drugs, such as aspirin and ibuprofen
- Prescription corticosteroids, such as prednisone
- Prescription hormones, such as oral contraceptives
- Highly refined carbohydrates, such as candy bars, cookies, cakes, and soft drinks
- Mold and fungi found in grains, fruits, and refined carbohydrates

Currently, the best way to identify leaky gut syndrome is to monitor symptoms. People who have the condition can help themselves by taking digestive enzymes with every meal, taking probiotic supplements daily to correct any imbalance among beneficial and harmful bacteria in the gut, steering clear of foods to which they're sensitive, and limiting the consumption of fatty foods, caffeine, and alcohol.

MALNUTRITION

Chronic severe malnutrition can also cause sensitivities. If people are deficient in protein, vitamins, and minerals, the enzymatic and metabolic processes that the body requires for efficient functioning cannot occur. This can result in undigested food and an increase in toxic metabolites, which can eventually lead to sensitivities. Vitamins and minerals are also needed for effective immune function, which protects the body in fighting off infections.

DRUGS

Chemotherapeutic drugs, excessive use of antibiotics or steroids, or exposure to toxic chemicals or radiation are important factors in developing sensitivities or depressed immune reaction. For example, when antibiotics and steroids are used concurrently over a long period of time, as is often the case with asthmatics, the antibiotics destroy the good microflora of the intestines, thereby strengthening and increasing the longevity of bad microflora, or yeast, which can lead to candidiasis. A suppressed immune system is unable to destroy these yeast cells, which can eventually scar the intestinal villi (which help it absorb nutrients). This allows toxins, undigested food, and yeast to enter the bloodstream through the intestine, leading to a systemic yeast problem.

Types of Sensitivities

Sensitivities can be classified according to the causative substance or the resulting symptoms. There are also active (acute) sensitivities and hidden (chronic) sensitivities.

The first category of sensitivities, defined by their causative substances, includes the following subtypes:

+ Ingestants, also referred to as food sensitivities
+ Injectants, such as drugs
+ Insect sensitivities
+ Inhalants, such as dust
+ Contactants, such as latex or chemicals
+ Infectants, such as viruses or bacteria
+ Physical agents, such as cold or heat
+ Organs
+ Autoimmune sensitivities, such as being sensitive to one's own hormones, including thyroid, estrogen, testosterone, cholesterol, and adrenaline

The second category of sensitivities are those that can be defined by their symptoms. These include

+ Skin conditions, such as eczema, hives, and rashes
+ Anaphylaxis
+ Hay fever
+ Asthma
+ Headaches and migraines
+ Stomach upset
+ Chronic fatigue
+ Depression
+ Chronic pain
+ Conjunctivitis
+ Sensitivity-related diseases

Active or acute sensitivities can be of the "immediate type," in which symptoms appear within seconds of contact after every exposure (for example, hives, itching, vomiting, coughing, or wheezing), and they usually subside within an hour. Or they can be of the "delayed type," in which the reaction occurs hours or days after contact. For example, some food sensitivities are not to the food itself, but to a chemical by-product of digestion.

Hidden or chronic sensitivities may cause serious developmental and functional problems or deficiencies and chemical imbalances. For example, a sensitivity to B vitamins can cause B vitamin deficiencies and result in chronic health problems, such as chronic fatigue syndrome, attention deficit hyperactivity disorder (ADHD), depression, digestive problems, asthma, and headaches. This book will focus on the diagnosis and treatment of chronic sensitivities.

SENSITIVITIES DEFINED BY THEIR CAUSATIVE SUBSTANCES

The following sections describe sensitivities defined by their root cause. They are organized in order of importance, with the most common sensitivities, which are most crucial to BioSET clearings, at the beginning.

Food Sensitivities

Ingestants are items taken in by the mouth, such as solid foods and beverages. A food sensitivity is the immune system's response to a certain food, which occurs when IgE-mediated chemicals trigger a sensitivity reaction. After ingesting foods to which a person is sensitive, they may experience vomiting, stomach pain, swelling and bloating, diarrhea, constipation, eczema, hives, an asthmatic attack, breathing difficulties, joint pain, migraines, and, on occasion, anaphylaxis. In extreme cases, the food is not ingested and an individual has a sensitivity reaction to minute amounts of the allergen, such as skin contact with the food or kissing someone who has eaten the food.

The seven types of foods that cause 90 percent of all food sensitivity reactions are

1. Milk

2. Eggs

3. Wheat

4. Tree nuts, especially peanuts

5. Soy

6. Fish

7. Shellfish

Peanuts, nuts, fish, and shellfish commonly cause the most severe and dangerous reactions.

Children and adults with food sensitivities experience a wide variety of symptoms, including abdominal pain, headaches, runny noses, asthma, chronic coughing, attention problems, and behavioral problems. While it is generally believed that these sensitivities will disappear as a child matures to adulthood, in reality they do not. Often some of the acute symptoms lessen over time, but the sensitivity becomes chronic or hidden, potentially causing developmental or functional problems and persistent maladies.

While up to 25 percent of adults believe that they have food sensitivities, conventional medicine claims that only 1 or 2 percent actually do! Those who do not have sensitivities, according to the limited definition used by mainstream medicine, have what is called a "food intolerance," which can be equally uncomfortable. Essentially, the difference between the two labels is this: a genuine food allergy is caused by antibodies that can be identified by blood testing, while a food intolerance is a broader term encompassing many illnesses caused by food. A food intolerance does not register on conventional allergy tests though it can be measured using muscle testing.

Some causes of food intolerance (sensitivity) are chemicals such as caffeine and food colorings such as tartrazine, which do not produce adverse effects in the majority of the population, but do trigger sensitivity symptoms in some people. A deficiency of enzymes (the chemicals that help digestion) can cause problems as well. If a person lacks one or more digestive enzymes, they may experience digestive problems like diarrhea and stomach pain after consuming the food the missing enzyme normally digests. For example, many people who have difficulty drinking milk have lost the enzyme that digests lactose, the sugar in milk. In my clinical practice I have also found that some of these people who are "lactose intolerant" are actually sensitive to lactose. When we clear for lactose using BioSET, they are fully able to tolerate milk, with no side effects.

Studies indicate that taking antibiotics can increase the chances of food intolerance in some people. The antibiotics apparently kill some types of bacteria in the large intestine and allow others to flourish, causing an abnormal reaction during digestion that produces various unpleasant chemical by-products and associated symptoms. Antibiotics can also cause abnormal amounts of yeast or candida (a fungus that can cause yeast infections) in the intestines, which can lead to an imbalance of other healthy intestinal flora or microorganisms. I have had successful results in clearing candida and other abnormal pathogens with BioSET.

Drug Sensitivities

A small percentage of people experience a severe, even life-threatening reaction to certain drugs and chemical additives, particularly penicillin. Other problematic drugs include aspirin, vaccines, insulin, and illegal drugs such as marijuana. Most often, the sensitivity reaction will appear as a skin condition, whether it is itching, hives, rashes, swelling, or peeling skin. Other symptoms may include incontinence, headache, dizziness, high blood pressure, moodiness, depression, agitation, edema, insomnia, hyperactivity, heart palpitations, bloating, constipation, diarrhea, blurred vision, hot flashes, and, of course, drug dependence and addiction. For example, five thousand men and women who participated in Operation Desert Storm experienced severe side effects, most likely sensitivity reactions to a pill they were instructed to take every day called pyristigimide bromide.[2] This drug was supposed to protect them from harmful exposure to nerve gas. After taking this substance, these men and women developed numerous health problems, from tearing eyes and runny nose to chronic fatigue, twitches, cramps, blurred vision, incontinence, diarrhea, and other serious maladies. Even now, fourteen years later, they continue to experience these symptoms, as well as to show signs of a suppressed immune function and long-term muscle damage.

Insect Sensitivities

In general, the normal toxic reaction and discomfort that follows an insect sting is not considered to be a sensitivity. However, many people have severe reactions to bee and wasp stings, which can sometimes be fatal. These IgE-mediated reactions induce rashes, running nose and eyes, swelling of the throat, asthma attacks, and anaphylactic shock.

Occupational Environment Sensitivities

Some people develop sensitivities as a result of working with industrial dusts, vapors, gases, fumes, and substances such as nickel, chromium, rubber, dyes, formaldehyde, or glues, or working in heat. Symptoms may show within weeks, or they may take years of repeated exposure to appear. The least-protected parts of the body—the hands, arms, and face—are the areas most frequently affected. Protective masks, gloves, and clothing can help prevent a reaction and even save a life. For example, bakers who handle different foods to which they may be sensitive, such as milk, eggs, and wheat flour, can prevent reactions by wearing gloves and masks if necessary.

Latex Sensitivities

Often categorized as an occupational environment sensitivity because it is frequently found among health care workers, a sensitivity to latex is surfacing among increasing numbers of the general population as well. Latex falls under the contactant category, since the sensitivity reaction arises from skin contact with the substance. The offending material can be found in balloons, gloves used for washing dishes or handling food, dental and medical gloves, condoms, clothing and shoes, carpets, rain slickers, pacifiers, baby-bottle nipples, and even air pollution. Symptoms include swelling, welts, itchiness and hives, sneezing and nasal congestion, watery and itchy eyes, chronic fatigue, and occasionally anaphylactic shock. Generally, people with the highest risk of developing latex sensitivity are those with high levels of exposure to latex, a history of sensitivities, multiple surgeries as children, or food sensitivities. In fact, studies have shown that people with sensitivities to certain fruits and vegetables—particularly bananas, kiwis, raw potatoes, tomatoes, celery, carrots, figs, avocados, papayas, passion fruit, hazelnuts, and water chestnuts—are more likely to develop latex sensitivity.

SENSITIVITIES DEFINED BY THEIR SYMPTOMS

The following sections discuss sensitivities as defined by the symptoms they cause. It includes the most common symptoms, listed in order of prevalence, with the most common symptoms at the beginning.

Skin Conditions

The most common skin condition, eczema, is a rash or irritation that can be either wet or dry, occasionally chapped, and most often accompanied by severe itching. Although the cause isn't always clear, the condition often appears in children of families with a history of sensitivity disease, so it may be hereditary.

With children, I usually find that eczema is caused by a sensitivity to vitamin C, wheat, corn, and B vitamins. In adults, the most common allergens are foods, clothing, animals, chemicals, creams, fungus, yeast, and bacteria. Milk and woolen clothes are possible contributors to the condition. Eczema usually begins in the first year of life as a facial rash and is often a precursor of asthma. Later in life it can appear on the insides of the elbows and the backs of the knees, and on the neck, ankles, wrists, and the backs of the hands. Contact eczema's symptoms are similar to those of common eczema, but they can be traced to direct contact with a variety of substances, including nickel found in coins, stainless steel, chromium found in cement and leather, rubber found in gloves and boots, and preservatives found in creams, ointments, and cosmetics.

Hives, or urticaria, is experienced as a warming of the skin along with redness and itching or white, raised wheals. It can appear very suddenly and may last for hours or a whole day.

Anaphylaxis

The most severe and life-threatening allergic reaction, anaphylactic shock, also called anaphylaxis, is usually brought on by a sudden immune response to foods, insect stings, or medication. Symptoms—which include swelling, difficulty breathing, hives, vomiting, diarrhea, cramping, and a drop in blood pressure—can occur in as little as five to fifteen minutes. Immediate medical attention is needed when a person goes into anaphylaxis, so call 911. While waiting for medical assistance, stimulation of the respiratory acupuncture points may provide some relief of the symptoms and improve breathing. Refer to the emergency treatment procedures in the BioSET chapter of this book.

Hay Fever (Allergic Rhinitis)

Hay fever, also called allergic rhinitis, is a condition that afflicts millions of Americans. Symptoms include a runny or stuffy nose, sneezing, swelling of the mucous membranes, loss of smell and taste, and itchiness of the throat, palate, and eyes. Primary causes are airborne inhalants, such as grass, weed, or tree pollens, and mold spores. Hay fever can be seasonal or intermittent.

Asthma

During an asthma attack, an individual's bronchial tubes will swell, and the muscles surrounding the tubules will go into spasm. This obstructs the flow of air to the lungs, leading to wheezing, coughing, and difficult, labored breathing. Asthma may begin at any age and has the potential to recur and become chronic. It is always triggered by allergens, including foods, pollens, environmental factors such as perfume, animal dander, chemicals, bacteria, climatic conditions, and emotions such as stress. When these sensitivities are active from birth, asthma may be recognized early in life, even in infancy. When these sensitivities are hidden and chronic, they may cause other chronic functional and developmental problems, such as fatigue, coughing, or headaches. Hidden and chronic sensitivities are difficult to detect because tissues break down slowly, with minimal secretion of immune mediators, causing only minor muscle contractions, swelling, and increased mucus secretion. However, when other stressful factors are added to the system—

for example, menopause, emotional stress, medication use, or gastritis—the sensitivity load on the body is increased and late-onset asthma may occur.

Sensitivities and Chronic Illnesses

We usually don't imagine that sensitivity reactions play a role in seemingly unrelated medical conditions. However, many experts are drawing connections between a history of sensitivities and numerous other chronic conditions, from alcoholism to obesity. Sensitivities are even considered partially responsible for some types of behavioral or emotional problems. In my practice I have had excellent results treating obesity, ADHD, mild and moderate depression, and exhaustion, since I know that these problems are likely to be rooted in sensitivities, digestive stress, and toxicity. Once the basic sensitivities are cleared using BioSET, these conditions either improve or resolve completely.

ALCOHOLISM

The idea behind treating alcoholism by desensitizing the body is based on the fact that many alcoholics are sensitive to the ingredients in alcoholic beverages and, therefore, cannot digest them. A person who has a sensitivity to a certain type of food, such as the fruits and grains from which alcohol is brewed and the sugars that make up a large part of these beverages, is deficient in those nutrients, leading to strong cravings. While alcoholics may think that they feel better when they are drunk, they are actually caught in a vicious cycle. Substances to which they may be sensitive include B vitamins, sugar, grapes, brewer's yeast, malt, or corn. As a result, they become addicted to an alcoholic beverage that contains the allergen.

I have cleared alcoholics successfully with BioSET. Alice, a woman in her thirties, had been an alcoholic for ten years. During this time she had been involved in some near-fatal car accidents and some financial disasters due to her drinking. Although she had tried a number of treatment facilities and therapists, none of them had been successful in curing her. She hoped that I might be able to help her with her intense craving for alcohol, which would then enable her to make better progress with her behavioral treatments.

I performed a full BioSET evaluation on Alice, which included a complete enzyme and detox evaluation and a sensitivity testing. Like most alcoholics, Alice was especially sensitive to the B vitamins and sugars found in alcohol. As I said earlier, people usually crave the foods to which they are sensitive. I prescribed an enzyme for sugar digestion and began to clear her from the first sequence of sensitivities, which included the B vitamins and sugars. Then I cleared Alice for alcohol. Six hours after the treatment, she called to tell me she was drunk. I immediately felt disappointed. But then she added that she was drunk not on alcohol or sugar, but simply as a result of the process of clearing the sensitivity. She was cognizant of everything that was happening, which was never the case when she was really drunk. She was detoxifying from the alcohol. She also noted how good she was feeling.

The next day, when I retested Alice, she was no longer sensitive to alcohol. Directly afterward, she checked into a three-week alcohol treatment program. Three years later I received a call from her telling me how grateful she was for all my help. She said she hadn't had a single drink since the sensitivity clearing, which was indeed a breakthrough for her.

OBESITY

Like alcoholics, people who struggle with excessive weight gain may be sensitive to their favorite foods; therefore, they are unable to resist indulging their intense cravings. In addition, some people have noticed that hunger can be a symptom of a sensitivity reaction. For example, when someone with a sensitivity to wheat eats a wheat-heavy meal, they may feel strong cravings to eat again within a short period of time, even though they no longer need the nutrition. This is referred to as reactive hypoglycemia.[3]

A fifty-year-old woman recently came to the BioSET clinic for help with her weight issues. A very well known nutritionist in Los Angeles, she had tried every possible diet and weight loss regimen with no success. No amount of commitment to following a diet seemed to help. She had heard of BioSET and food sensitivities, and she wondered if eating food she was sensitive to could be the root of her own inability to lose weight. We evaluated her for food sensitivities and began desensitizing her to the foods that were healthy and on her good diet regimens. In the beginning, her weight loss was modest, a couple of pounds here and there. But this was better than nothing, so she continued. After three months of desensitizing and coming to the clinic once every three to four weeks, the weight began to drop. She is now 14 pounds lighter and is very delighted.

ARTHRITIS

In some people, arthritis can be partially attributed to a sensitivity reaction to common foods, causing swelling and pain in the joints. For this reason, when some arthritic patients avoid certain foods or environmental allergens, their symptoms diminish. Acidic foods (refer to chapter 7) seem to be especially troublesome, as are plants and vegetables from the nightshade family, which include tomatoes, white potatoes, eggplant, peppers, and tobacco. I have also found arthritic patients to be sensitive to bacteria and parasites, which can trigger an autoimmune or autoaggressive reaction.

A woman named Nancy, who suffered from severe arthritis of her sacroiliac and hips, came to see me seeking help with her extreme chronic pain and migraine headaches. She was a professional housekeeper and cook, which required her to be active and on her feet most of the day. When I performed a full examination and sensitivity testing on Nancy, I found her to be highly sensitive to all the basic allergens, including acid-forming foods, the nightshade family, and fifteen different types of bacteria. She was unable to digest proteins and fats, yet she was eating large amounts of protein because she was trying to lose weight. The uric acid content in her urine sediment was quite high, which is generally an indicator of high protein consumption.

I recommended an enzyme to help Nancy digest fats and proteins, and I prescribed a diet lower in protein and fats and higher in complex carbohydrates. I then cleared her with the BioSET desensitization for all of her sensitivities, including the acidic foods and the bacteria. After all the bacteria were cleared, her hip and sacroiliac pain almost completely subsided and her flexibility improved by 75 percent. In addition to being able to take care of her household responsibilities, she now walks three miles a day and has lost thirty pounds. She also smiles a lot when I see her!

MIGRAINES AND OTHER HEADACHES

Sensitivities are a common culprit in recurring headaches. Research studies have shown again and again that some migraine sufferers can eliminate their symptoms by avoiding certain triggering foods, particularly milk, eggs, wheat, aged cheese, MSG, chocolate, oranges, tea, coffee, beef, corn, cane sugar, yeast, and alcoholic beverages.[4]

A sensitivity to smoke, exercise, pollen, chemical fumes, and stress can also cause chronic headaches.

Nancy, my arthritis client, also experienced headaches every day, as well as weekly migraines. No remedy she had tried had worked for her headaches. While clearing her for arthritis, I also cleared her for female hormones, such as estrogen, progesterone, thyroid hormones T3 and T4, and adrenaline. I had to clear Nancy for progesterone three times before her sensitivity completely cleared. I also taught her to clear herself at home for this sensitivity, since it was such a severe sensitivity for her. After completing her hormone clearings, Nancy's headaches disappeared and have never returned.

Psychological and Behavioral Effects of Sensitivities

Perhaps some of the least recognized but most interesting effects of sensitivities are psychological conditions. Evidence is mounting that in some people certain allergens can actually result in, or aggravate, emotional and behavioral problems, including depression, hyperactivity, learning difficulties, anxiety, irritability, and schizophrenia. BioSET practitioners have had excellent results with attention deficit disorder, hyperactivity, and other behavioral problems in both children and adults. Children with ADHD are cleared for the basic sensitivities, plus possibly mercury and fluoride; thyroid hormones; yeast or candida; foods, such as wheat, dairy, sugar, artificial sweeteners, food additives, food coloring, and chocolate; environmental sensitivities, such as radiation, dust, chemicals, mold, and pollution; and emotional traumas. The children then supplement their diet with digestive enzymes and an enzyme mineral formula. Treating children with BioSET is fulfilling and rewarding because the changes in their physical and emotional health are immediate and profound.

Testing for Sensitivities

In addition to self-assessment questionnaires, which can help you determine whether you have the symptoms commonly associated with various sensitivities, there are a number of frequently used sensitivity tests that a qualified health professional can administer to evaluate your sensitivities: skin reaction tests, blood tests, a pulse test, muscle testing, and electronic testing.

Self-Assessment Questionnaires

The following self-assessment questionnaire will help you determine whether you have the symptoms that commonly raise the suspicion of having sensitivities. If you reply with six or more "yes" answers, it would be a good idea to undergo further testing and/or consult with a doctor.

1. Do any of your blood relatives suffer from sensitivity syndromes (such as hay fever, asthma, skin rashes, or severe reactions to drugs or insect stings), food sensitivities, addictive disorders (such as alcohol or drug abuse or compulsive eating), diabetes or low blood sugar, arthritis, headaches, or digestive disorders? Were any of your blood relatives hyperactive, learning disabled, or bed wetters as children?

2. Did your mother experience severe stress during her pregnancy with you? Was your birth difficult or complicated?

3. As an infant, did you have any problems tolerating bottle formula or breast milk? Did you have problems with gaining weight, colic, or spitting up?

4. As an infant, did you suffer from frequent digestive, respiratory, or skin problems?

5. Were you "difficult" in infancy and/or childhood, often crying or irritable? Were you overactive or underactive? Did you have problems sleeping, or trouble learning or paying attention at school?

6. As a child, were you often sick, plagued by ear infections, sore throats, swollen glands, colds, bronchitis, croup, stomach aches, constipation, diarrhea, or headaches?

7. As an adult, are you always tired, even though you get enough sleep?

8. Do you frequently have puffy eyes? Wrinkles or dark circles under your eyes? Itchy, red, watery, burning, painful, or light-sensitive eyes? Blurred vision? Baggy, swollen eyelids?

9. Do you often have a stuffy, watery, runny nose? Do you sneeze several times in a row? Rub your nose upward or wiggle your nose? Do you have one cold after another, without feeling sick? Nose bleeds? Excessive mucus?

10. Do you have asthma or suffer from wheezing? Do you cough or wheeze with laughter, with exercise, with cold air, with cold drinks, or at night when it's damp outside?

11. Do you have skin rashes, such as eczema or atopic dermatitis? Itchy rashes or hives, especially in the creases of your arms or legs? Cracked toenails or fingernails? Acne? Dandruff? Loss of hair?

12. Do you have recurrent earaches? Fluid behind your eardrums? On and off hearing trouble? Ears popping or ringing? Flushed, red earlobes? Dizziness? Itchy ears? Drainage from your ears?

13. Do you suffer from digestive problems? Swelling or soreness of your face and lips? Itchiness on the roof of your mouth? Canker sores? Bleeding gums? Bad breath? Nausea and stomach aches? Excess gas, diarrhea, and/or constipation? Belching? Itchy rectal area? Ulcers? Colitis?

14. Do you have difficulty gaining or losing weight?

15. Do you have repeated bladder infections, difficulty urinating, and/or water retention?

16. Is your pulse or heartbeat irregular after eating?

17. Have you ever had seizures?

18. Do you have sinus problems, earaches, or sore throats? Headaches, dizziness, convulsion? Insomnia? Leg or muscle aches, back pain, swollen or stiff joints, arthritis? A constant low-grade fever, a feeling of being flushed or chilled, excessive sweating, fainting spells?

19. Are you a picky eater? Do you indulge in binge eating?

20. Do you feel like you are high one moment and low the next, with depression appearing for no reason?

21. Do you have trouble concentrating, sometimes feeling confused and spacey? Or are you hyperactive, overly nervous, frequently anxious, and/or quick to anger?

22. Does a change in your surroundings or the seasons affect how you feel?

If you are an asthmatic, here is a set of questions to determine whether or not you are in complete control of your asthma. Developed by the Asthma Zero Mortality Coalition (AZMC), they are known as the Asthma Alert. If you answer "yes" to four or more questions, you require additional help to get your condition under control.

1. Have you gone to the emergency room more than once in the last year for treatment of your asthma?

2. Have you missed more than one day of school or work in the last year due to asthma?

3. Have you been awakened more than once in the last month by coughing or wheezing?

4. Have you seen your doctor at least once in the past six months for your asthma?

5. Does asthma keep you from participating in certain sports or exercises?

6. Are you using more than one canister per month of any of your bronchoinhalers?

7. Are you using your inhaled bronchodilator more than three or four times a day?

8. Do you sometimes forget, or choose not, to take your prescribed asthma medication?

9. Do you feel you could use more instruction on how to properly use your inhaler?

10. Does your peak flow meter indicate airflow obstruction?

To help you further assess the extent of your asthma, here is another helpful questionnaire developed by the American College of Allergy, Asthma, and Immunology. If you reply with six or more "yes" answers, it would be a good idea to undergo further testing and/or consult with a doctor.

ACTIVITIES

1. When I walk or do simple chores, I have trouble breathing or I cough.

2. When I perform heavier work, such as walking up hills and stairs or doing chores that involve lifting, I have trouble breathing or I cough.

3. Sometimes I avoid exercising or taking part in sports like jogging, swimming, tennis, or aerobics because I have trouble breathing or I cough.

4. I have been unable to sleep through the night without coughing attacks or shortness of breath.

SYMPTOMS

5. Sometimes I can't catch a good, deep breath.

6. Sometimes I make wheezing sounds in my chest.

7. Sometimes my chest feels tight.

8. Sometimes I cough a lot.

TRIGGERS

9. Dust, pollen, and pets make my asthma, cough, or trouble breathing worse.

10. My asthma gets worse in cold weather.

11. My asthma gets worse when I'm around tobacco smoke, fumes, or strong odors.

12. When I catch a cold it often goes to my chest.

HOSPITAL VISITS

13. I made one or more emergency visits due to asthma or breathing problems in the last year.

14. I had one or more overnight hospitalizations due to asthma or breathing problems in the last year.

MEDICATION PROBLEMS

15. I feel like I use my asthma inhaler too often.

16. Sometimes I don't like the way my asthma medicine(s) make me feel.

17. My asthma medicine doesn't control my asthma.

ANXIETIES

18. My breathing problem or asthma controls my life more than I would like.

19. I feel tension or stress because of my breathing problem or asthma.

20. I worry that my breathing problem or asthma affects my health or may even shorten my life.

Skin Reaction Tests

Some tests for allergies involve provoking a sensitivity reaction in the skin through exposure to a minute amount of an allergen. Most commonly, this is accomplished by applying drops of an allergenic extract to the skin surface, which has been pricked or scratched. This is called a scratch test. Other skin reaction tests include

- Introducing a small quantity of allergenic extract between the layers of skin with a needle (called an intradermal test)
- Placing a piece of gauze soaked in a suspected allergen over the skin for a prolonged period of time (called a patch test)
- Putting a drop of allergenic extract in the eye (called a conjunctival test; this is rarely used today)

If the test is positive, the site of the injection or exposure will swell and the surrounding area will become inflamed. This is generally not useful in determining food intolerance, but it is a simple method of detecting sensitivity to inhalant allergens. A reaction may occur after as little as fifteen minutes or not until fifteen hours later.

Blood Test (RAST)

The radioallergosorbent test (RAST) is an initial lab test that is administered to a single blood sample. Blood tests measure the amount of IgE antibodies in an individual's blood. This is an important indicator since the more allergic the individual, the more these antibodies increase. The blood sample is tested for specific IgE antibodies against likely allergens in the patient's area of residence.

Pulse Test

Pulse testing for sensitivities, which measures the heart rate before and after exposure to a suspected allergen, is an effective method for determining sensitivity reactions to foods. While pulses can be felt at various points throughout the body, the most common and simplest pulse to locate is the radial artery at the wrist. To take this pulse, lightly place three fingers over the artery on the inside of the wrist, slightly above the thumb. Other areas to read the pulse are the temporal region of the skull (by the front temples), the popliteal region (the indentation in back of the knee), the pedal pulse (the area behind the ankle bone), and the carotid artery in the neck. A normal pulse should beat evenly and forcefully, at a regular rhythm, with no delays, interruptions, or other irregularities.

When a person is sensitive to the allergen being tested, the pulse generally will deviate from normal. It usually becomes faster and more forceful, but it can also become slower and weaker. For this reason, a pulse test can be helpful in detecting a food sensitivity. Unfortunately, if one eats several foods at a time, which of course we all do, it is hard to determine exactly which food is causing the sensitivity reaction. Many of my patients have come into my office already knowing they have food sensitivities because they used this method of diagnosing.

Muscle Testing

Also known as applied kinesiology, muscle testing was developed in 1964 by Dr. George Goodheart, a chiropractor, to diagnose or read energetic blockages in the body. He used the relative strength of the muscles to uncover structural misalignments in the body, for chiropractic care purposes.

Muscle testing can also be used to discover sensitivities in the body for the treatment of allergies, which will be discussed in further detail in chapter 10. Here are the basics: The person to be tested either lies down or sits up. He then extends one arm at a ninety-degree angle, thumb down, in front of him. The facilitator pushes against his arm to establish the basic strength of the person's muscle, the "indicator muscle." When the test subject holds a food or other substance to which he is sensitive, the indicator muscle will immediately and noticeably weaken to the point where it becomes easy to push down the subject's arm, even when he is trying hard to keep it extended. These procedures can detect both hidden sensitivities and active, or acute, sensitivities, identifying which substances should be avoided.

SURROGATE MUSCLE TESTING

Surrogate muscle testing can be used to determine sensitivities in infants, young children, and elderly, weak, or physically incapacitated adults. It utilizes energy conductivity to diagnose sensitivities in a person who otherwise could not be muscle tested. A surrogate touches the person being tested, and the facilitator muscle tests the surrogate. When the actual person being tested holds a particular item, the surrogate's response indicates whether that person has a sensitivity to the item.

O-RING TEST

People can test themselves using the O-ring test, similar to muscle testing. The person makes a circle by opposing their little finger and thumb on one hand. Then with the index finger of the other hand, the person tries to separate the two opposing fingers. Initially, the thumb and little finger making the circle should be strong and inseparable. If they are not strong, there may be a structural misalignment or carpal tunnel syndrome, which may render this self-testing technique ineffective. If the circle is strong, the next step is for the person to hold the potential allergen in the hand they are testing, with their remaining three fingertips touching the allergen. If the little finger-and-thumb circle remains strong when the other index finger pulls on it, they are not sensitive to the substance. However, if their fingers weaken when tugged and the circle separates, they are sensitive to the substance.

This technique takes practice to learn, but it can be a survival tool for severely sensitive individuals, who can use it to test suspect foods before eating them.

Electronic Test (EAV)

Electronic devices have been used for more than a century in treating and diagnosing patients. Dr. Reinhard Voll, a German medical doctor and dentist, believed the body is comprised of energetic roadways or conduits that flow throughout the entire system in specific pathways called meridians. Together with fellow German scientist Fritz Werner, they designed and built an electronic instrument to chart and verify the relationship of acupuncture points to the corresponding organs and systems. This instrument, an EAV, or electro acupuncture meter, can directly infer the functional status of these systems.

The EAV method causes little or no discomfort, as there are no needles and the skin is not punctured. The patient holds a brass handle in one hand, and a metal probe is placed against acupressure points on the hands and feet. A doctor or technician charges the specific acupuncture points with approximately one volt of direct current. A reading is taken for each point along particular meridians. The readings show any "irritation" to the electromagnetic pathways or organ systems (that is, blockages to the flow of electromagnetic energy) by reading the person's galvanic skin response, which is a measure of the flow of energy.

Other electronic devices like the one developed by Voll are used to test for food and environmental sensitivities. Correlations with other testing procedures have shown that the EAV test is quite accurate in detecting sensitivities to foods, chemicals, pesticides, herbicides, environmental irritants, dental irritants, fungus, bacteria, and viruses, as well as dysfunctions of organs and systems.

Electromagnetic Testing for Medications

In the mid 1970s Dr. H. Roy Curtin, a physicist directing a variety of research projects at Eyring Research Institute in Utah, was asked to evaluate EAV, which was being used in Europe to test medications. During a demonstration of their technique, Voll and Werner had discovered that the value of an electrical measurement at an acupuncture point was influenced if the person being evaluated held a bottle containing an appropriate medicine, but not when holding an inappropriate medicine.

This led to the practice of searching for appropriate medications that would help restore balance in the acupuncture meridians. Researchers did this by having a client repeatedly hold different medicines and then using a meter to remeasure the acupoint until a medicine was found that produced a shift in the reading, that is, an appropriate medicine.

Other doctors made a similar discovery, observing that they could detect a change in a muscle's strength response when a subject held an appropriate medication in their hand. For example, often when a person holds artificial sugar, their arm strength is weakened when tested. (Many people are very sensitive to artificial substances.)

In both cases, the medicine being tested was contained in a sealed container. The person did not have to take the medicine in order to produce the effect either on the acupoint or the muscle. This ruled out the skin absorbing the medicine and causing a direct chemical action. Therefore, it was originally supposed that the effect must be the result of some sort of electromagnetic interaction between the medicine and the subject. At first researchers assumed that the effect was the result of electromagnetic frequency resonance, analogous to the science of radio reception. However, this model turned out to be inadequate to explain the very real and observable phenomenon of appropriate medicines, sealed in containers, triggering physical responses.

In addition to his extensive theoretical and experimental research in electromagnetism, Dr. Curtin was involved at the time with a variety of U.S. government research projects designed to explore the range of human capabilities. Based on the findings of these studies, he proposed the hypothesis that even though the observed response could not be explained on the basis of chemistry or electromagnetism, nevertheless it demonstrated that humans have the ability to discern the contents of sealed bottles and that this ability could be used to develop a safe and highly effective procedure for screening candidate medications.

Versions of this technology have been successfully used by thousands of practitioners worldwide for almost thirty years now. For those who are skilled in its use, there is no system of equal accuracy in the diagnosis and resolution of complex individual health issues.

Rotation Diets

Rotation and elimination diets, also called exclusion or simplification diets, are widely used by physicians and individuals both to diagnose and to eliminate sensitivity reactions. These regimens remove all potential allergens from the diet and then reintroduce them one at a time at different intervals while observing their effects. Although they can be helpful in detecting hidden sensitivities, rotation diets are difficult to sustain and generally fail. It may be efficacious to introduce some foods to which you are sensitive on a rotation basis for a period of time after being cleared with BioSET.

Types of Sensitivity Treatments

Of course, the simplest and most effective approach to treating sensitivities is to avoid the allergenic substance entirely. However, when avoidance is difficult or even impossible, as with environmental allergens, a number of other treatments are available. Let's take a look at some of these treatments.

Medications for Sensitivities and Asthma

Medication is probably the most commonly used treatment for sensitivities, and there are a vast number of medicines in use today. There are antihistamines to relieve itching, hay fever, and irritation from airborne allergens; bronchodilators or inhalers for asthmatic symptoms; decongestants; steroids; corticosteroids; and a drug called cromolyn, which is taken orally before eating to prevent gastrointestinal symptoms. Used primarily to suppress symptoms, these medications can have many side effects, including drowsiness, anxiety, frequent and painful urination, nausea, dry mouth, vomiting, loss of appetite, abdominal discomfort and cramps, constipation or diarrhea, headaches, loss of sexual libido, depression, and fatigue.

Among asthma medications, which are designed to reverse the irritation and constriction of air passages in the lungs and bronchial tubes, there are two main types:

+ Relievers, or bronchodilators, which are designed to relax the muscles in the bronchial tubes and provide rapid relief of asthma symptoms. The relievers include beta-2 medications, anticholinergics, and theophyllines.

+ Preventers, which are designed to reduce inflammation in the airways and prevent asthma symptoms. The preventers can be either steroids or nonsteroids.

RELIEVER MEDICATIONS

The most widely used reliever medications in the treatment of asthma are the beta-2s, which include salbutamol, orciprenaline, fenoterol, terbutaline, and procaterol. Although they are usually taken through an inhalant device known as a puffer, they can also be administered as tablets or syrups. The beta-2s provide immediate relief that lasts up to four hours. The oral preparations provide longer-lasting relief but can cause side effects, in particular, a fine tremor of the hands or slight heart palpitations. Beta-2 medications are extremely effective in treating acute asthma episodes.

PREVENTER MEDICATIONS

Preventer medications work to reduce inflammation, congestion, and "twitching" in the bronchial tubes. Steroids, the most powerful preventers available today, may cause a yeast infection, which can lead to soreness and white spots in the mouth and throat. When taken for long periods of time, steroid medications may suppress the body's natural production of steroids, reduce growth rate, cause weight gain, diabetes, or cataracts, and weaken bones. However, short courses of steroid tablets (prednisone) are extremely effective in treating acute asthma episodes.

Cortisone, a steroid, is used in treating acute sensitivities. But cortisone can have serious side effects, causing severe stress on the immune system, and can create other serious health problems, from osteoporosis to chronic fatigue. Studies have shown that debilitating effects can appear after a single dose, and permanent damage can set in within weeks of starting treatment.

There are three nonsteroid preventers, each of which acts in a slightly different way. These medicines are safer, but supposedly less powerful than the inhaled steroids and are more frequently used with children.

COMMON ASTHMA MEDICATIONS

There are currently 281 asthma medications available. Here is a list of some of the most commonly used ones and some information about them.

Generic Name: Budesonide (Brand Name: Pulmicort Turbuhaler, Pulmicort Respules)

HOW DOES IT WORK?: Budesonide, a preventer, is a human-made glucocorticoid steroid related to the naturally occurring hormone cortisol (hydrocortisone), which is produced by the adrenal glands. Used in an inhaler, these glucocorticoid steroids have powerful anti-inflammatory effects that reduce inflammation and spasming of the airways caused by asthma. The budesonide works by going directly to the inner lining of the inflamed airways.

WHO USES IT? This drug should be used by individuals who require continuous, prolonged treatment. This includes people who experience frequent asthma attacks requiring a bronchodilator or those who have nighttime asthmatic episodes.

Budesonide can be prescribed for persons six or older, but it should not be used to treat an acute asthma attack. While some effects might be observed within twenty-four hours, maximum effects may not be seen for one to two weeks. Doses vary widely. Adults usually administer one to four puffs, twice daily. Children usually receive one to two puffs, twice daily. For people with mild asthma, once a day may be sufficient.

ARE THERE SIDE EFFECTS? The most common side effects are mild coughing or wheezing, which can be minimized by using a bronchodilator inhaler such as albuterol (Ventolin) prior to using budesonide. Oral candida or thrush (a fungal infection) may occur in one out of twenty-five people using this drug, especially in the higher doses. The risk in children is lower than in adults. Hoarseness or a sore throat can also occur in 10 percent of users, but it can be minimized by using a spacer device. Washing out your mouth with water following each use reduces your risk of thrush and hoarseness. In less common cases, alterations in the voice may occur.

Generic Name: Flunisolide Inhaler (Brand Name: Aerobid)

HOW DOES IT WORK? Another preventer, this medication is a corticosteroid, which acts in the lungs to reduce inflammation resulting from chronic asthma. It is breathed into the lungs using a special inhaler. If using other inhalers, wait several minutes between uses and then inhale Aerobid, the corticosteroid, last. This medication is best used at even intervals, usually once in the morning and once in the evening. Do not increase your dose or stop using this medication without first consulting your doctor.

WHO USES IT? Adults can use flunisolide. Caution is advised when administering this drug to children since there is a slight chance that it will slow down their growth. However, it should not affect their ultimate height as an adult.

Before beginning use of this drug, make sure your doctor has your complete medical history, including all of your illnesses and infections, your recent exposures to contagious diseases, and any conditions you may have such as glaucoma, cataracts, and allergies, especially drug allergies.

ARE THERE SIDE EFFECTS? You may experience a dry or irritated throat, hoarseness, or coughing while your body is adjusting to this medication. If any of these symptoms continue or become bothersome, inform your doctor. Call your doctor if you develop any unusual symptoms, such as a rash, sore throat, mouth sores, swelling of your face, wheezing, breathing trouble, or changes in your vision.

WARNING: If you switch from an oral corticosteroid such as prednisone tablets to this inhaler within a twelve-month period, or if you use this product in higher-than-usual doses and then suddenly quit using it, your body may have stopped producing enough natural steroids. In this case, you may need to begin taking oral corticosteroids, especially if your body is fighting a major infection or recovering from surgery or some type of injury. Under these circumstances, call your doctor immediately if you experience unusual weakness, sudden weight loss, or dizziness.

Generic Name: Salmeterol (Brand Name: Serevent)

HOW DOES IT WORK? In asthmatics, the accumulation of mucus, muscle spasms, or swelling of the airway lining can narrow the breathing passages, leading to shortness of breath, wheezing, coughing, and congestion. Medicines used to open airways in asthma patients are known as bronchodilators. Salmeterol, a reliever, is a bronchodilator of the beta-2 agonist type, a medication that stimulates beta-2 receptors on the muscle cells lining the airways, causing these muscle cells to relax, opening the airway and easing breathing.

Allergens such as pollen can cause the airway to narrow; they stimulate the mast cells, a class of immune cells located around the airways, to release histamine. Histamine, a chemical known as an immune mediator, is excreted by the body in allergic reactions and causes symptoms such as congestion. Salmeterol blocks the release of histamine by the mast cells, thus preventing the airway from narrowing when exposed to allergens.

WHO USES IT? Salmeterol should be used twice daily (morning and evening) by individuals twelve or older to help control asthma and prevent spasm of the airways. This medication can also be used to help prevent exercise-induced asthma attacks. Salmeterol is a long-acting beta-2 agonist that begins working within fifteen minutes and can last more than twelve hours. This medication is generally not recommended for patients whose asthma symptoms can be easily controlled with the infrequent use of short-acting inhalers.

ARE THERE SIDE EFFECTS? This medication's side effects include accelerated heart rate, palpitations, elevated blood pressure, tremor, nervousness, headaches, and irritation of the throat and upper airways.

Generic Name: Fluticasone Propionate and Salmeterol Oral Inhaler (Brand Name: Advair Diskus)

HOW DOES IT WORK?: Advair Diskus, both a reliever and a preventer, is a bronchodilator used to open airways and decrease inflammation in those suffering from asthma. Advair Diskus contains a combination of salmeterol, a bronchodilator of the beta-2 agonist type, and fluticasone propionate, an anti-inflammatory corticosteroid. Beta-2 agonists are medications that attach to beta-2 receptors on the smooth muscle cells that surround the airways, causing the muscle cells to relax and open the airways. Fluticasone propionate is a human-made glucocorticoid steroid, which is related to the natural hormone cortisol. In asthmatics, fluticasone propionate suppresses inflammation within the airways, reduces the muscle spasms that narrow these airways, and reduces swelling and mucus. In lower doses, very little fluticasone is absorbed into the body. However, in higher doses, the drug is absorbed and may cause side effects.

WHO USES IT? Advair Diskus is used to control asthma in people twelve years of age and older who require continuous treatment. This includes individuals who experience frequent episodes of asthma that require bronchodilators or who have nighttime episodes. This drug goes into effect within half an hour to an hour, and the benefits can last more than twelve hours. Advair Diskus is generally not prescribed for patients whose asthma can be controlled easily with infrequent administration of short-acting inhalers. Advair Diskus should not be used to treat acute episodes of asthma. This drug is used twice daily in the morning and evening.

ARE THERE SIDE EFFECTS? Between 20 and 25 percent of those using this medication experience upper respiratory tract infections. Approximately one out of eight people experience headaches as a side effect.

Generic Name: Triamcinolone Acetonide Inhaler (Brand Name: Azmacort)

HOW DOES IT WORK? Triamcinolone acetonide is a human-made steroid and a potent anti-inflammatory, a preventer. When used as an inhaler, this medication goes directly to the airways of the lungs, and very little is absorbed into the body. It is usually administered in the form of a 100 mcg per actuation inhaler.

WHO USES IT? Triamcinolone acetonide is prescribed to control bronchial asthma in individuals who require continuous treatment, including those who experience frequent asthma attacks requiring bronchodilators or those who experience asthmatic episodes at night. This drug is used to prevent asthma attacks and should not be used to treat acute (active) attacks.

ARE THERE SIDE EFFECTS? The most common side effects are mild coughing or wheezing, which can be minimized by using a bronchodilator inhaler such as albuterol (brand name, Ventolin) prior to using the triamcinolone acetonide. Oral candida or thrush (a fungal infection) may occur in 5–10 percent of people using this drug, especially with higher doses. The risk in children is lower than in adults. Hoarseness can also occur, but it can be minimized by using a spacer device. Washing out your mouth with water following each use reduces your risk of thrush and hoarseness.

Alternative Treatments for Sensitivities and Asthma

All of these asthma drugs have allowed many people, children as well as adults, to live relatively normal lives, and they have saved thousands, if not millions, of lives. But they do not get to the root of the asthma and enable these individuals to free themselves of their dependence on medication. In contrast, BioSET does get to the root of asthma by assessing and clearing the sensitivities that cause and trigger the asthma. By detoxifying, restoring digestion with enzyme supplements, and desensitizing the asthma sufferer to each of these sensitivities, BioSET can reduce or occasionally completely eliminate the need for medication. In chapters 4–7, I will explain the many sensitivities that can trigger asthma, and in chapter 9, I will describe an effective technique for clearing these sensitivities. The following options are alternatives to traditional medicines that can help to alleviate sensitivity reactions.

IMMUNOTHERAPY

Allergy shots, or immunotherapy, are another commonly used treatment approach. Allergy shots desensitize the person to the allergen by injecting a small amount of an extract of the substance under the skin's surface. The dose is gradually increased until a maintenance dose is obtained. After three years, once the allergy has been eliminated, the injections are generally stopped.

Allergy shots are often effective in treating allergies to pollen, dust, and animal dander, but they have not proven useful with food allergies. In addition, food shots may cause side effects, including sore arms, hives, throat spasms, and on occasion even death. By controlling reactions to airborne allergens, however, shots can reduce the load effect and thereby reduce the allergic response to foods.

For many years, doctors have tried using allergy shots, primarily for pollens, to treat people who suffer from asthma attacks. Studies have shown that while these people were receiving the shots, they suffered fewer asthmatic symptoms, but the effects diminished over time and disappeared entirely after two years. In addition, these shots are extremely expensive.

HOMEOPATHY

Homeopathy is a natural health system that is based on the concept that like cures like. It uses minute doses of a remedy that would usually produce disease-like symptoms to cure a disease. Homeopathic treatment appears to have a positive effect in treating sensitivities in asthmatics and people with other disorders related to food and environmental sensitivities. A study carried out at Bristol Homeopathic Hospital in the United Kingdom on homeopathy revealed that more than 70 percent of patients with chronic diseases said homeopathy helped them feel better. The six-year study involved over 6,500 patients. And 89 percent of those with asthma said homeopathy helped them.[1] Many people report positive effects with homeopathy, but there have not been many studies, other than this one. BioSET utilizes homeopathy for detoxification with excellent success in helping reduce symptoms with asthma and allergies.

EPD

Enzyme-potentiated desensitization (EPD) is a method of immunotherapy that Dr. Leonard McEwen of London developed in the mid 1960s. It desensitizes the patient by using a series of injections that contain a combination of mixed allergens and the enzyme beta-glucoronidase, administered every two to three months at first and then less frequently over time. Because many allergens are treated at once, only nine or ten injections are required, and the results are reportedly longer lasting than with conventional allergy shots. Beta-glucoronidase in combination with other allergens causes T suppressor cells to multiply and differentiate and causes them to recognize the allergen originally injected. These T cells then supposedly suppress any adverse reaction when one is then exposed to these allergens.

EPD is not widely available in the United States due, in part, to the FDA's restrictions of importation. Development of low-dose antigens (LDAs) has been started as a potential replacement that could become available soon. However, I do not know how successful this approach has been for asthma.

BEE POLLEN

An anti-sensitivity product that has gained some popularity in recent years is bee pollen, which is actually a mixture of bee digestive enzymes, nectar, and reproductive dust from the flowers visited by the bees. Because bee pollen contains some of the airborne grass and ragweed pollens to which people are most sensitive, it can act as allergy shots do by desensitizing an individual with a small quantity of the substance to which he or she is sensitive.

The difference, however, is that allergy shots deliver pollen in an undiluted form, whereas oral dosages get broken down by enzymes during the digestive process. What this means is that, to achieve the same results, a patient might have to take up to ten thousand times as much pollen orally as they would receive through an injection. The other disadvantage of taking bee pollen is that one never knows exactly what it contains, since it varies from week to week and from beehive to beehive. Also, bee pollen in large dosages can cause unpleasant side effects, such as nausea or stomach upset.

CHIROPRACTIC CARE

Chiropractic care has been known to help strengthen the immune system by strengthening the nervous system. A healthy immune system means resistance to disease, sensitivities, and chronic illness. A healthy nervous system is one that is free of spinal musculoskeletal misalignments. Chiropractic practices suggest that skeletal imbalances, particularly in the spine, can lead to the loss of nervous system integrity and, hence, to the loss of health elsewhere in the body.[2] Many studies have observed the effect of a healthy nervous system on immune system health.

In particular, chiropractic care has proven effective with asthmatics in restoring nerve supply to the lungs and bronchioles and helping to feed and restore the respiratory system.

ACUPUNCTURE

Extensive research has shown that acupuncture can help people with a variety of conditions, including pain, anxiety, arthritis, eczema, migraines, and sensitivities, by promoting natural healing and improving bodily functions. Developed and practiced in China over the past two thousand years, acupuncture treats the whole person, rather than just a particular disease. It attempts to address the root cause of a problem rather than symptoms alone and works to restore balance between a person's physical, emotional, and spiritual well-being. Instead of treating standard points for specific sensitivities, the acupuncturist will treat each sensitive individual differently, depending on the diagnostic picture that emerges after examining the pulses, the tongue, and other indicators.

Acupuncture has proven successful in reducing the sensitivity of allergic individuals. For example, in the December 1993 issue of the *Journal of Traditional Chinese Medicine*, acupuncture and desensitization were compared in the treatment of 143 cases of individuals with IgE-immune antibody allergies. The results proved that acupuncture therapy had a remarkable action against these allergic reactions. The curative effect was higher in the acupuncture group with allergic asthma, allergic rhinitis, and chronic hives. [3]

Emergency Treatment

In the event of anaphylactic shock or other emergency due to extreme sensitivities, it is crucial that the patient receive first aid treatment within the first ten to fifteen minutes. People who are prone to severe allergic reactions should carry a kit with antihistamines and an injection of the drug epinephrine (a bronchodilator that opens the airways and restores blood pressure to normal) for immediate emergency self-treatment. If an individual is severely allergic to insect stings, applying a tourniquet near the sting will slow the circulation and absorption of the venom into blood. Placing ice on the sting area can reduce swelling.

A patient in anaphylactic shock should lie on their side with their head turned to the side to avoid choking should they need to vomit. If the person stops breathing, mouth-to-mouth resuscitation should be performed by someone who knows how to do it. As soon as possible, the person should be taken to a hospital emergency room or doctor's office.

PART TWO

Asthma: Warning Signs, Symptoms, Respiratory Diseases, Causes, and Preventive Measures

| CHAPTER 4 | # What Is Asthma? |

Asthma is a respiratory condition that affects more than twenty million Americans and is one of the leading causes of school and work absences. Additionally, one in every twenty children is affected by this disease. In the past years, despite advances in medical treatment and medication, the incidence of asthma among women and children has increased and the number of fatalities due to asthma have risen over 50 percent. The number of new cases and the yearly rate of hospitalization for asthma have also increased: 25 percent of emergency room visits in the United States are related to asthma.[1]

In asthmatics, the bronchial tubes overreact, being hypersensitive and hyperactive; therefore, it is also called wheezy bronchitis or bronchial asthma. When an asthmatic's bronchial tubes are temporarily narrowed or blocked by mucus, breathing becomes difficult.

During an asthma attack, the muscles around the airways tighten, the linings of the airways become inflamed and swollen, and the glands produce an overabundance of thick mucus, further narrowing the airway passages. The asthmatic has difficulty breathing, especially exhaling carbon dioxide, which means that the body has less oxygen available and carbon dioxide can build up to dangerous levels. Once an asthmatic has suffered an asthma attack, triggered by some substance or condition, the airways in the lungs become sensitive to other triggers, which results in chronic asthma, or the manifestation of more symptoms.

Asthma Can Be Life Threatening

While most people have heard of asthma, few realize how serious or life threatening it can be. One patient that I had successfully treated for asthma with BioSET had a forty-seven-year-old friend who was also an asthmatic. She frequently suggested that her friend come to see me, but due to various circumstances, the woman never did.

One weekend the friend went to Las Vegas. While she was in a casino, she started to have an asthma attack, probably triggered by smoke, alcohol, or food sensitivities. Unable to locate her inhaler, she collapsed and died. Because the security guard and the people around her did not realize what was happening to her, they could not help.

Recognizing an Asthma Sufferer: Warning Signs of Asthma

There are many different warning signs of asthma. For that reason, it is important for people to learn how to recognize their own red flags and take appropriate actions. Most sufferers have one or more of the classic symptoms, which include the following:

+ The first symptom is wheezing accompanied by a whistle when breathing. The whistle can range from hardly noticeable to quite loud.
+ The second symptom is coughing, a mild cough or a hack that just will not stop.
+ The next classic symptom is chest tightness, similar to a tight grip around the chest.
+ The last symptom is shortness of breath. People with this symptom cannot take a deep breath. They feel as if they are trying to breathe through a straw, or worse, like they are drowning. Exhaling is especially difficult.

Pulmonary function studies, such as those done with a spirometer, are breathing tests that can accurately measure lung capacity. A person breathes into a closed tube that is connected to a machine that shows how well the person is breathing. These machines determine how much air a person can blow out and how much their lungs can hold. Asthmatics have difficulty exhaling due to obstructed bronchioles.

SIGNS OF ASTHMA IN CHILDREN

If a child has had several bouts of wheezing, shortness of breath, or coughing, he or she probably has asthma, particularly if the symptoms come and go. The child may wake up frequently at night coughing and wheezing because symptoms tend to worsen at night. In infants and young children, asthma is often difficult to distinguish from chest infections such as bronchitis. Therefore, doctors may prescribe antibiotics or cough syrups but, typically, the symptoms will not respond to those sorts of treatments. Depending on the child's age, the symptoms may interfere with feeding, exercise, and even speech, and a teacher might send a child home often because of frequent coughing that disrupts the class.

In young children, asthma is a likely diagnosis if recurrent head colds with coughs and wheezing occur several times a year and persist for several weeks. Many physicians will ask questions about symptoms to determine which factors, such as infection, exercise, or sensitivities, bring on the symptoms. Usually, the doctor will take an allergy and sensitivity history when it is clear that the asthma is caused by sensitivities to certain substances. In fact, most people diagnosed with asthma are also diagnosed with sensitivities. It is important for a doctor to note whether a child responds to antiobiotics or to asthma medications.

The Happy Wheezer

The "happy wheezer" is a term used to describe a baby aged three to twelve months who develops a wheeze that may persist for weeks or even months. These infants are active and not distressed. They feed well and gain weight well. Sometimes they do not require treatment, and their wheeze settles down in the second year of life. Usually it is related to certain allergens, such as breast milk, fabric, or feathers.

Testing Children for Lung Function

Since the main problem in asthma is a narrowing of the bronchial tubes, doctors have developed lung function tests to measure how much the tubes have narrowed from their standard size. These tests can be used to diagnose asthma. The tests are simple and painless and can usually be done easily by children over five or six. However, they cannot be used by younger children.

The simplest of these tests checks the peak flow rate with a device called, not surprisingly, a peak flow meter. In this test the child is asked to breathe in deeply and then blow out as hard and fast as possible through the meter, as if blowing out a candle. The meter then measures the maximum speed with which the child can force air out of the lungs, or the peak flow rate. If the bronchial tubes are blocked, the child cannot achieve a normal speed. This is called a reduced flow rate. Asthma medication dilates the bronchial tubes to allow more air to flow. If a child responds well to this medication, this confirms a diagnosis of asthma.

The exercise test is also quite simple. The child runs on a treadmill or rides a bicycle for six minutes, and the peak flow rate is measured before, during, and after exercise. Most children with asthma will show a drop in the peak flow rate after exercise.

The challenge test uses a chemical called methacholine, which causes a slight narrowing of the bronchial tubes in children with asthma but has little or no effect on those who do not have it. In this test the lung function is measured, the child is asked to inhale a mist of methacholine, and the lung function is measured again. The strength of the methacholine is gradually increased and the lung function test repeated until the bronchial tubes narrow and lung function begins to fall slightly. This test gives a measure of the bronchial tubes' degree of sensitivity and how much they are affected. The smaller the amount of chemical needed to cause a narrowing of the airways in the lungs, the greater the sensitivity, which means the child has asthma.

The challenge test is safe and painless, and the child is closely observed throughout the procedure. Because children under five are not able to do reliable breathing tests, diagnosis in that age group is usually based on symptoms and how patients respond to asthma medications and antibiotics.

In 1995 the American College of Allergy, Asthma, and Immunology announced a simple and inexpensive screening test to help with the early detection and management of exercise-induced asthma. Called the free-running asthma screening test (FRAST), it involves measuring the breathing of high school students, having them run for sixty-seven minutes nonstop, and then testing them again. Studies using this test have found a 13–18 percent incidence of exercise-induced asthma, including students who did not know they had asthma.[2]

A major advantage of this kind of test is that gym teachers or other school personnel can give them to large groups of students. The objective is to make asthma screening tests as routine as hearing tests. A disadvantage of the FRAST is that some children might not be able to run for sixty-seven minutes. Also, because results may vary depending on seasonal factors like humidity and temperature, the test must be repeated at different times of the year. Despite these limitations, the FRAST is one of the best methods available to diagnose subtle asthma in high school students and prevent it from becoming life threatening in the future. Subtle asthma requires testing for diagnosis because its symptoms are not as obvious as those of full-blown asthma.

HOW TO RECOGNIZE SIGNS OF AN ASTHMA EPISODE IN YOUR CHILD

It is especially important to learn the signs of an asthmatic episode in children. Adults will usually recognize when they are having or are about to have an asthma attack, but children may not. For this reason, their parents need to be able to detect the danger signs and get treatment when necessary. Early signs include increased coughing at night or early in the morning, more breathlessness with exercise, an increased need for bronchodilator medicine, and a decrease of 20 percent or more in peak flow readings below the child's personal best value.

There are four signs that tell a parent when a child is getting into trouble with asthma:

+ The first sign is a high-pitched whistling wheeze at night that is more pronounced as the child breathes out. As an asthma episode progresses, the airways will be blocked and the wheezing will stop. This is a sign of a worsening condition.

+ The second sign to watch for is retractions in the chest wall, where the soft tissue is sucked in as the child inhales. These are most obvious below the rib cage, and parents will also notice that the child uses the large muscles in the neck to help breathe.

+ The third sign of asthma is prolonged exhalation. Because the bronchial tubes are blocked in acute asthma, a child has difficulty getting air out of the lungs. As a result, exhalation becomes prolonged and labored.

+ Finally, during an acute episode, the child usually becomes short of breath and therefore may have difficulty putting words together or be unable to sleep or exercise. Normal breathing rates will also increase.

Precursors of Asthma

People who develop asthma first get eczema, which is an itchy skin condition that manifests in early infancy. Eczema will usually affect the cheeks of infants and the elbow and knee creases of older children. Children with eczema usually are sensitive to C and B vitamins, which indicates, or may be a precursor to, a fruit and/or wheat sensitivity. When these sensitivities are cleared with BioSET, the eczema usually clears up readily, and the later occurrence of asthma is prevented. Eliminating B vitamin sensitivities is also necessary for eliminating sugar sensitivities, which is important for overall good health.

Eczema has been described as the "itch that rashes." It is characterized by an intense itching that provokes scratching and keeps the skin chapped. Sometimes it oozes, and it can become infected. Chronic scratching can lead to a dry, scaly, and thickened skin known as lichenification. Atopic (hereditary) dermatitis is usually caused by allergens, including foods, heat, wool or other clothing, animals, feathers, wheat, milk, eggs, soy, peanuts, and fish. Clearing for the appropriate allergen with BioSET can make atopic dermatitis or eczema disappear.

Some children with asthma, or with sensitivities that have the potential to develop into asthma, also have allergic rhinitis, an irritation of the lining of the nose and eyes that produces a runny nose, sneezing, and red, itchy, watery eyes. Asthma can be prevented in these children by clearing the sensitivities causing the rhinitis.

Symptom Complexes of Asthma

Asthma can develop at any age. About 25 percent of children with asthma develop symptoms in their first year of life. While asthma varies greatly from one person to another in terms of how severe the symptoms are and how often they occur, most people fit into one of four basic types: mild, moderate, severe, and coughing. Each of these types has specific treatment needs.

MILD ASTHMA

Those who suffer from mild asthma have normal breathing tests unless they are currently displaying asthmatic symptoms. The frequency of attacks follows three basic patterns. Approximately 30 percent have mild symptoms only once or twice a year. (These are infrequent occurrences.) Another 30 percent have mild, intermittent symptoms of asthma (less than two episodes a week) with normal breathing tests. A final 30 percent have mild, persistent symptoms of asthma (two or more episodes a week) with normal breathing tests. Mild persistent asthmatics may require daily preventative medications. For example, they may be on inhaled corticosteroids as well as bronchodilators.

Because their symptoms clear up quickly with the use of bronchodilators, most people with mild asthma use medications only when needed. As for causes of this type of asthma, mild cases are most commonly triggered by viruses and viral sensitivities. Some people only have symptoms seasonally when the pollen count is high.

Mild asthma symptoms can be relieved almost entirely, and very quickly, by clearing a few basic sensitivities. Children or adults who are just beginning to show signs of becoming asthmatic can be cleared for the basic allergens and then treated for specific allergens like pollens or viruses with great success.

MODERATE OR SEVERE ASTHMA

Forty percent of asthmatics have moderate or severe, persistent (daily or continuous) symptoms of asthma with abnormal breathing tests. This group requires daily preventative medications and must use a bronchodilator three to four times a day to maintain reasonable control of their condition, and they are admitted to the hospital frequently. Wheezing and coughing occur most of the time, and exercising and sports are difficult for them.

These people benefit from treatment for their basic sensitivities, but they need BioSET to clear many other sensitivities as well (see chapter 9). With the elimination of each sensitivity, they experience more freedom and fewer asthmatic reactions. While these patients may require up to a year of clearing with BioSET, home self-clearings may expedite the process. Dietary recommendations and therapy with the correct enzymes can usually reduce their use of medications within the first eight months.

COUGHING ASTHMA

One of the more difficult types of asthma to diagnose is coughing, or cough-variant, asthma. Often doctors will treat children with this form of asthma for bronchitis, colds, or allergies since all three of these conditions can cause coughing. However, these treatments won't stop the coughing for long, if at all. In coughing asthma, typically a cough is the sole or most predominant symptom. Individuals don't normally get wheezing or shortness of breath with asthma in its cough-variant form. The cough tends to be dry and typically gets worse at night, and individuals may use asthma medications to control it. I have found that this type of asthma is triggered by exercise, viral sensitivities, and infective sensitivities. Though coughing is not usually recognized as asthma, it is common in people of all ages. Some of these individuals develop the more typical symptoms of asthma later in life, and some do not.

Coughing asthmatics respond very well to BioSET since this condition is usually caused by sensitivities—most commonly to inhalants, perfumes, chemicals, fabrics, and infections—especially if there is mucus in the chest or a loose cough. When mucus is not present, this type of asthma is usually related to food sensitivities. Once a practitioner starts clearing a coughing asthmatic with BioSET, they stop coughing after eating certain foods.

One woman I treated coughed each time she ate chocolate. Apparently, her family had eaten an excessive amount of chocolate when she was a child. After I cleared her for chocolate, she never had the symptom again. Chocolate is a common asthma trigger, along with gas exhaust, gas heat, hormone supplementation, your own adrenaline (exercised-induced asthma), and atmospheric conditions.

Another patient, a young boy who came to see me, had suffered since the age of two from a chronic cough that was not related to any kind of infection. When he was cleared for some of the initial basic allergens as well as for sensitivities to wheat, corn, and bacteria, the cough stopped and he no longer had trouble sleeping.

A "BARKING" COUGH

Researchers are now studying another chronic cough, one that is involuntary or psychogenic. This cough usually has a "barking" or "honking" sound and can persist for months or years. The person may cough as often as every few seconds. This condition differs from asthma in that there is no shortness of breath, there is usually no difficulty conversing, and the cough disappears when the person is sleeping. Many of the tests are negative for any kind of pulmonary problem.

Allergic (Extrinsic) and Nonallergic (Intrinsic) Asthma

Whether mild, moderate, severe, or coughing, your doctor may refer to your asthma as being "extrinsic" or "intrinsic." Extrinsic, or allergic asthma, is more common (90 percent of all cases) and typically develops in childhood. Eighty percent of children with asthma also have documented sensitivities to certain substances. Typically, there is a family history of sensitivities. Additionally, other conditions, such as hay fever or eczema, are often also present. Allergic asthma often goes into remission in early adulthood. However, in 75 percent of cases, the asthma reappears later.

Intrinsic asthma represents about 10 percent of all cases. It usually develops after the age of thirty and is not typically associated with sensitivities. This type of asthma is more frequent among women, and many cases seem to follow upon a respiratory tract infection. The condition can be difficult to clear and symptoms are often chronic and year-round.

Conditions Related to Asthma

Some conditions and their symptoms are frequently associated with asthma. Here is a brief discussion of the more common types.

CHRONIC BRONCHITIS AND CHRONIC SINUSITIS

Chronic bronchitis and chronic sinusitis are the respiratory diseases or problems associated with asthma. Asthma sufferers usually have chronic bronchitis throughout the year, although it is more common during the colder, wetter months when they are more vulnerable to infection. These infections may be caused by infectants that are allergens themselves, or they may be linked with allergens, for example, cold, dust, or some foods. When these other allergens are encountered, the infectants (bacteria, virus, or fungi) can surface and create an infection that may lead to bronchitis or chronic coughing. Asthmatics must be cleared for these chronic infectant sensitivities with BioSET and enzyme therapy to break this linked reaction and rid themselves of these infections.

Up to 50 percent of all patients with asthma also suffer from chronic sinusitis, which can aggravate an asthmatic condition and produce asthmatic episodes. The symptoms of sinusitis are headache and tenderness of the sinus areas, as well as nasal congestion, postnasal drip, and stuffiness. The nasal congestion may worsen at night when lying down, resulting in coughing. Other symptoms include pain and pressure in the teeth, cheeks, forehead, and behind the eyes; fever; sore throat; earaches; bad breath; and a decreased sense of smell. Many different allergens can cause chronic sinusitis, including viruses, bacteria, inhalants, fabrics, pollen, dust, flowers, and perfume. Because people with chronic sinusitis end up with frequent earaches and chronic sinus infections, it can be especially important to treat for bacterial and viral sensitivities. If the infections are treated with antibiotics only, they will keep occurring. With BioSET these episodes can be prevented.

Over the years BioSET practitioners have had good results with a special cranial technique for people with chronic sinusitis. Called the nasal specific, it involves inserting latex balloons into the nasal passageways and inflating them, thereby opening the passages and allowing for drainage. It also rebalances and frees up certain cranial structures. Recently, EENT (eye, ear, nose, and throat) physicians have implemented a slight variation of this procedure, called balloon sinuplasty, under anesthesia, for chronic sinusitis.[3]

One man came to me suffering from chronic, sensitivity-related sinus headaches, which he had experienced his whole life. He had never had a sense of smell or taste, and he was subject to ongoing sinus infections, for which he was constantly taking antibiotics. He also complained of depression because of his tiredness and irritability and because he was unable to breathe, smell, or taste. I treated him with BioSET for a period of six to eight months, clearing all of his food sensitivities, such as wheat, dairy, and wine, and his sensitivities to viruses and bacteria. I also prescribed detoxifying homeopathics and enzymes. Because this man worked in a furniture factory, I cleared him for dust, wood, and upholstery, as well as for grasses and trees. Gradually, he regained his sense of taste and smell, and his sinus headaches and chronic infections disappeared.

When he came in for his last treatment, he said, "I never believed I could ever smell and taste. This has been a miracle. I have also seen incredible changes in my work. I have become more productive and successful. The people I work with say I am much easier to work with. I am happier, and my business has been booming ever since. Besides saving my life as far as changing my way of living, this has changed my work and allowed me to climb to new levels in my profession."

ALLERGIC RHINITIS, CHRONIC SINUSITIS, AND CHRONIC EAR PROBLEMS

Allergic rhinitis produces an itchy, runny nose, sneezing, nasal congestion, itching eyes, tearing, and red eyes. Some asthmatics have seasonal rhinitis caused by pollens in the spring, late summer, and early fall. Others have chronic, year-round rhinitis, which can lead to headaches and chronic congestion. Often related to sensitivities to indoor allergens such as house dust, molds, and pets, chronic rhinitis is characterized by stuffiness, mucous discharge, and nasal breathing problems when exposed to air-conditioning, heated houses with low humidity in the winter, weather changes, irritants, fumes, odors, or tobacco smoke.

When the sensitivities are linked to infectants, this condition can develop into chronic sinusitis as well as into complications such as sinus disease in the large tonsils, adenoids, sleep disturbances, otitis media (middle ear infection) and other ear problems, or middle ear disease. Children with allergic nasal disease are often restless sleepers who wake up at night because of coughing, a stuffy or runny nose, and sneezing. They have a thick nasal discharge, which is sometimes green. As the condition worsens, they may suffer headaches and fever, eventually developing asthma or causing their asthma to worsen. Other complications of allergic rhinitis may include the loss of taste and smell, resulting in decreased appetite and weight loss; oral facial deformities; nosebleeds; and teeth grinding.

Studies have shown that exposure to allergens may lead to the buildup of fluid in the ear and may obstruct the eustachian tube, which protects the middle ear cavity, drains secretions produced in the middle ear, and ventilates the middle ear.[4] Ear problems, chronic infections, and fluid in the ear can lead to hearing loss and a delay in speech development in children. More studies are needed to establish the relationship between substance sensitivity, ear infection, and fluid buildup in the ear, but there is enough information to determine that individuals with ear problems usually show signs of sensitivity to certain substances. They have a swelling of the nasal lining, nasal stuffiness, dark circles under their eyes, asthma, and eczema. There is a higher incidence of ear infections and fluid in the ear among children who live in places with many sensitivities, especially in homes where tobacco is smoked.

Many over-the-counter drugs do not help to prevent ear infections or fluid in the ears, but practitioners have had excellent results with BioSET. When there is fluid, many physicians use tubes to drain the ears, but this involves some risk of injury, as well as discomfort and inconvenience. Such invasive treatment is unnecessary because the chronic sensitivities related to ear infections and fluid in the ear can be cleared and eliminated with BioSET.

EMPHYSEMA AND BRONCHIECTASIS

Emphysema is a disease that is characterized by distended and damaged bronchioles and alveoli, by breathlessness on exertion, and by wheezing. Bronchiectasis is a disease that is characterized by dilation of the bronchi and the production of large amounts of sputum. A person with bronchiectasis has recurrent fevers and episodes of pneumonia; this condition may develop out of pneumonia or whooping cough. Both of these conditions can be characterized as bacterial sensitivities and may show some improvement when the patient is cleared for sensitivities to infectants, environmental toxins, inhalants, and food. Thus, while BioSET does not cure emphysema or bronchiectasis, it can help with the asthmatic symptoms that often accompany these ailments.

Environmental Causes of Asthma

Environmental sensitivities to substances such as chemicals, perfumes, pollens and other surrounding irritants can affect asthmatics more often and more severely than normal individuals. As a result, their breathing may be compromised.

Infectants

Infectants are at the root of severe asthma and often act as a trigger for asthmatic attacks. As a result, most of my clinical research in recent years has been in the area of infectants as allergens. Sensitivities to these infectants, including bacteria, viruses, fungi, and parasites, are common and can be debilitating.

BACTERIA

In a study that supports my theory of the link between infectants and asthma, David Hahn, MD, Medical Director of the Dean Foundation for Health Research and Education in Madison, Wisconsin, found that antimicrobial therapy can cure asthma in some adults who test positive for the bacteria *Chlamydia pneumoniae*. He found that 85–100 percent of the adult onset asthmatics in the study tested positive for C pneumonia bacteria, compared with only 50 percent of the general population.[1] Previous studies of antibiotic treatments may have been unsuccessful because they did not treat effectively for this organism. In my practice I have found a high incidence of this bacteria (bacterial sensitivity) in asthmatics and have had success clearing it with BioSET and enzyme therapy. Dr. Hahn contends that, despite doubts expressed by some experts, there is a growing body of evidence that bacterial sensitivities do exist.

PARASITES

Sensitivities to parasites like malaria or giardia can challenge and compromise an immune system. These parasites may live in the body for fifteen or twenty years and can be carried by children as well as adults. Children need to be taught to wash their hands after touching animals, because animals carry many parasites that can be passed on. Asthmatics can have sensitivities to parasites that lodge in the lungs. And a recent study discusses the increased likelihood of inflammation when parasites are present in the lungs. Chitin is a component of parasites and insects, and chitinases are produced in lower life-forms during infections with parasites and insects. Although chitin itself does not exist in humans, chitinases are present in human genes. It has been shown that in an asthmatic with sensitivities to parasites, the immune system does contain mammalian chitinase (AMCase) in exaggerated quantities. AMCase may be an important mediator (distributor) of asthma.[2]

FUNGI

Fungi sensitivities are another group of infectants that can cause chronic illness, particularly asthma and upper respiratory tract infections. These fungi include candida, aflatoxin, aspergillis, and many others. I rarely see an asthmatic who does not have fungi in their system, including candida. Candida is a systemic fungal infection that can manifest in different parts of the body. With asthmatics, it is sometimes found in the bronchus or lungs and may be a cause of emphysema. Candida can be cleared with BioSET and a ten-day diet, as discussed in chapter 11.

VACCINES

I include vaccine sensitivities in the category of infectants because they can be a troublesome trigger for asthma and other chronic health problems. BioSET practitioners have successfully cleared many children suffering from the side effects of diphtheria, pertussus, and tetanus (DPT) vaccines. When the DPT vaccine is given to people who are sensitive to it, it can cause a reaction that may trigger asthma. BioSET can successfully clear these sensitivities to the vaccines, rendering the vaccination harmless.

Several studies have been done in the United States and abroad on anaphylactic reaction to the measles, mumps, and rubella (MMR) vaccine to determine whether the reaction is caused by a sensitivity to eggs. A recent study reported that 222 children with severe egg sensitivity were safely immunized, and the majority of the handful of children who had an anaphylactic reaction to the vaccine did not have a history of egg sensitivity.[3] Researchers suspect that something else in the vaccine is causing the reaction. Perhaps the children are sensitive to the vaccine itself, which is why muscle testing is recommended.

I receive questions from parents regularly on whether or not they should immunize their children. It is a personal decision that each parent needs to make after careful study and research. A great deal is written about it.[4] I do recommend testing the children for vaccines before they are immunized to avoid adverse reactions. Reactions to vaccines can occasionally cause long-term health problems, especially for an asthmatic.

Adults need to think about vaccinations too. Every year many Americans receive a flu vaccine. When people ask me whether they should get vaccinated, I suggest that they be tested and cleared with BioSET to ensure they are not sensitive to the vaccine before they receive it. If people are sensitive to the vaccine, they can suffer many side effects, such as the flu, depression, sleeping problems, other central nervous system effects, muscle aches, fever, and flu-like symptoms. When practitioners clear their clients with BioSET for the flu virus, they rarely get the flu—and if they do, they only get a mild case.

The flu vaccine is produced from egg and activated particles of influenza viruses. For this reason, people with a strong sensitivity to eggs could react severely and should consider alternatives such as other flu prophylactic mediations and/or complementary supplements. Unfortunately, many people are not aware of their egg sensitivities. One man who had multiple food sensitivities but did not know he was sensitive to eggs had a flu vaccination and was sick for days. I finally cleared him for his egg sensitivity, and many of the symptoms cleared up. Now he tests for a vaccine before getting one.

TREATMENTS

BioSET practitioners have found that people suffering from chronic bacteria sensitivities often suffer from arthritis. Those with bacteria and parasite sensitivities may suffer from chronic gastrointestinal problems. People who have ulcers or gastritis are sometimes suspected of having Heliobactor pylori,[5] which is a bacterium that seems to play a part in duodenal ulcers. It is also suspected of being involved in sensitivities and allergic reactions such as hay fever. Chronic viral sensitivities can result in chronic infections like Epstein-Barr, mononucleosis, and herpes, and people with sensitivities to infectants tend to have more frequent chronic fatigue.

BioSET practitioners have also found that infectants can be associated with other sensitivities—food, environmental sources, inhalants, and even other infectants. Exposure to associated sensitivities can result in chronic infections, which act as triggers for asthmatics. For example, a chocolate sensitivity in an asthmatic can be associated with a bacteria, similar to the way that ear infections can be linked with food sensitivities.[6] When the asthmatic eats chocolate, an infectious reaction results—fever, excess mucus, bloating, sweating at night, sinus infections, ear infections, runny nose—and this reaction can trigger the asthma.

I believe that many of the antibiotics and other drugs used to treat infectants only drive them deeper into the system, while masking the symptoms, weakening the immune system, and toxifying the body, especially the liver. When a person is not allergic or hypersensitive to an organism, the immune system can easily eliminate the organism or, in extreme cases, antibiotics can do the job. An infectant that is an allergen can stay in the body and then surface when the immune system is weak or overloaded. The overload may occur because of an overabundance of sensitivities, emotional stress, or a toxic system. This reemergence can produce cycles of chronic bronchitis, chronic ear infections, and chronic sinus infections.

Asthmatics tend to store many bacteria and viruses in their systems as sensitivities, creating excessive mucus, coughing, wheezing, sore throats, tightness in the chest, and difficulty breathing. Practitioners have found BioSET to be dramatically successful in both children and adults for treating infections of viruses, including flu and herpes; bacteria; parasites; and fungi, including candida.

Individuals can be successfully cleared with their own saliva at the first sign of infection, such as a runny nose, a cough, a slight fever, or tightness of the chest. This technique is particularly effective if they have already been cleared for many infectants, keeping in mind that new infectants are always showing up. I discovered this treatment when a colleague became ill with a cough, fever, and runny nose at a seminar we were attending. I cleared him with the BioSET desensitization for his own saliva and recommended a protease enzyme as well as a vitamin C enzyme formula (see chapter 13 for information on enzyme formulas). To my amazement he began to improve, and after the second treatment he was much better.

This incident began a research project in my practice and at home. As soon as one of my family members would sneeze, cough, or experience any symptoms, I would have them spit into a glass and conduct a muscle test on the saliva. If they showed any weak response, I immediately cleared them with the BioSET desensitization. Invariably they improved immediately, and their symptoms disappeared. Clearing with BioSET when symptoms first arise in combination with some systemic enzymes can instantaneously reverse symptoms and consequently prevent an asthma attack or further progression of an infection.

When working to clear a chronic illness such as asthma, it is important to check the person's saliva at the first signs of infection, while continuing to clear all other possible infectants to prevent further sensitivities. To help prevent asthma, I often clear asthmatics for their saliva on every visit in case they have been exposed to some new infectant.

Ingestants

Drugs, including vitamins, can also cause problems. Aspirin, for example, is a common trigger for asthmatics. One asthmatic client told me that she was at a party recently and got a headache. Someone helpfully gave her an Excedrin, and she immediately began wheezing and had to use her inhaler. Chemical dyes such as tartrazine, which are used in some foods and drugs, can also cause reactions.

When new patients come to see me, I always make sure they bring any drugs they are taking, including antidepressants such as Prozac, Zoloft, and Welbutrin and synthetic hormones such as Synthroid. Many people are sensitive to these drugs because they are synthetic chemicals that the body does not produce naturally. Occasionally and with caution, BioSET practitioners will clear drugs—which may need to be done over and over again and checked every few months, perhaps because the companies change some of the materials and a new prescription is not the same as the last—but this is only something advanced practitioners do and not something to be done at home with asthmatics. It is important to look at each drug as a potential sensitivity.

Inhalants

Inhalants are environmental allergens that we breathe. Although we often don't see them, they can do a great deal of damage. One of the most severe types of sensitivities for asthmatics, they can be handled easily with BioSET clearings. Some common sources of inhalants are listed below, in alphabetical order.

COCKROACHES

Cockroach droppings are a type of house dust. Tropical in origin, these common pests require a constant source of heat and, therefore, tend to infest buildings that are continuously heated. In contrast to dust mites, cockroaches are not affected by changes in humidity and are able to search for water in taps, drains, toilets, and even people's mouths. Since the two determinants of cockroach infestation are heat and food supply, it is not surprising that apartment houses and projects are particularly susceptible. Indeed, for inner-city children, cockroaches may be the major source of indoor allergens associated with asthma.[7]

COOKING FOODS

Allergens can be contained in the steam from cooking foods. Some people cannot even be in close proximity to food to which they are sensitive. One time I was clearing a young boy for sugar, and suddenly I noticed that his mother was about to pass out. "You know," she said, "sometimes even being near foods to which I might be sensitive brings on symptoms." She was feeling faint in reaction to the sugar that her son was holding.

In one study, researchers boiled shrimp and analyzed the steam. They found shrimp allergens in the steam and concluded that inhaling such steam may cause significant reactions in sensitive individuals.[8]

FEATHERS

Feathers can produce a variety of reactions. Many people sleep with down pillows and comforters, unaware that feathers may cause sinus problems and trigger asthma. One woman who came to me had experienced sinus problems most of her life. We cleared her for feathers with BioSET, and after twenty-five hours I retested her. Her runny nose and other sinus symptoms were completely gone.

HOUSE DUST

The worst indoor sensitivity for asthmatics is house dust. There are many components of house dust that may provoke sensitivity reactions, but the most important are dust mites. A dust mite is a microscopic insect-like creature related to the spider that lives in mattresses, pillows, blankets, carpets, upholstered furniture, and curtains. Carpeting laid over concrete tends to harbor dust mites. It thrives in humid and warm conditions and at low altitudes, and its diet consists of shed scales of human skin. Female mites can lay twenty-five to fifty eggs, with a new generation produced every three weeks. Mattresses and other household items contain large numbers of living and dead mites. The waste product of these creatures is the main sensitivity in house dust, and the one that causes the most problems for asthmatics. Each mite produces about twenty waste particles each day, and these particles can continue to produce sensitivity reactions, including runny nose, sneezing, watery eyes, coughing, and wheezing, long after the mite is dead.

Several studies have shown that children exposed to dust mites are more likely to become asthmatic. The allergens that the mites produce is so hard on the lungs that they can trigger asthma in some individuals. The level of exposure to house dust mite allergens and the severity of asthma in children are intricately linked.

House dust can also be produced indoors from fibers and plant and animal material in the home, such as feathers, cotton, wool, jute, hemp, or animal hairs, which are found in many household items. Less appealing components of house dust may include human skin scales, animal dander and saliva, molds, and cockroach droppings.

Jackie, an eight-year-old girl with asthma, would cough incessantly after going to bed every night. When we cleared her for dust, mattress, and upholstery sensitivity with BioSET, she no longer coughed at bedtime.

MOLDS

Molds are microscopic fungi made up of clusters of filaments. Unable to produce their own food from sunlight and air, they live on plant or animal matter that they decompose for their nourishment. Molds are some of the most widespread living organisms, with tens of thousands of different varieties. Bread mold may be the most familiar. Some molds are beneficial— they produce penicillin or other antibiotics, or are necessary for agriculture. However, others produce potent toxins or are major sources of plant disease. Many molds reproduce by releasing spores into the air that settle on organic matter and grow into new mold clusters. These airborne mold spores are far more numerous than pollen grains and can cause symptoms of mold sensitivity when inhaled.

Molds are found in most environments, indoor and outdoor, and on food. Their distribution varies from region to region. Unlike pollens, molds do not have a limited season, though their growth is encouraged by warmth and high humidity. As a result, they are more prevalent during humid seasons. Outside, molds are present in the air unless there is a cover of snow on the ground. They are most prevalent in shady damp areas, on decaying leaves and other vegetation, and where plant materials have been disturbed. The highest fungal levels are in temperate zones, near oceans, and in areas with the least snow cover.

In North America, grain crops are particularly susceptible to smuts and rusts. Farm workers exposed to these fungi often have many symptoms of sensitivity. Exposure is greatly increased by such activities as thrashing, bailing, and combining, which can release spores. People doing yard work spread spores as well when cutting grass or clearing dry brush. Peak levels for the spores of fungi such as alternaria and cladosporium are reached on hot, breezy, rain-free days. At night and during rainfall, a very different array of fungi is found. They are ascomycetes, fleshy types called basidiomycetes, and yeast, which require high humidity and splashing water droplets to become airborne.

Some molds are produced in humid areas of the house, such as bathrooms and basements, while others enter from outside. Houses are never completely free of mold, and exposure is high in areas where plant material has been stored or processed. Molds include mildew and rust, which is also an allergen. Molds also exist in our diet in such foods as blue cheese, along with the other member of the fungi group, mushrooms.

Molds are highly irritating to asthmatics; in fact, I have never known an asthmatic who is not affected by them. Molds can cause a stuffy or runny nose, sinusitis, nasal polyps, eczema, and many other kinds of problems. BioSET clearing for mold and mold spores can cause dramatic improvement in severe asthmatics, as well as in people with chronic health problems such as chronic fatigue and poor digestion. One woman I cleared suffered arthritic pain in her back every time she sat down on a particular piece of furniture. It turned out she was reacting to mold in a plant near the furniture.

PETS

Another common source of sensitivities is domestic pets. BioSET practitioners routinely clear people for sensitivities to animals and animal dander, including sheep wool and goose down. Cat dander is the most potent, and controlling the dander can be difficult. A cat carries 60 to 130 milligrams of allergen on its coat and sheds it at the rate of about .1 milligram per day. As a result, carpets and upholstered furniture can accumulate large quantities of cat dander. Removing the animal may be the most effective control measure, but the results will not be immediate. Allergens can remain in a house for months after an animal is removed.

Individuals with animal sensitivities can react to proteins from the animal's dander, urine, or saliva, which are spread throughout the house. The urine of small animals such as gerbils and mice also can produce allergic reactions and cause problems for asthmatics. In the case of cats, the allergy is produced by proteins in the dander and saliva, not by cat hair. The allergens become airborne as microscopic particles, which when inhaled into the nose and lungs can produce asthma symptoms. Although individual cats may produce more or less allergen, there is no relationship between the pet's hair length and allergen production, and there is no such thing as a nonallergenic breed of cat.

Cat allergen can even be found in homes where cats have never been and in office buildings or public places where animals are not allowed. This is because cat allergen is particularly sticky and is carried on clothing from places with cats to other locations. It is almost impossible not to be exposed to some level of cat allergen. Because more allergen is present in locations with cats, of course, a sensitive individual is more apt to have a rapid onset of symptoms there. The amount of airborne particles can be reduced by opening windows, using exhaust fans, and employing efficient air cleaners.

Carpets, upholstered furniture, and mattresses will hold cat allergen even after a cat is removed or banished from the bedroom. It can take up to twenty weeks for allergen levels in carpets to decrease to the level found in homes without cats, and up to five years in mattresses. Since cat allergen can also be found on vertical surfaces, walls should be cleaned as well when attempting to decrease allergen levels.

Because cat allergen is so potent and such a potential trigger for asthmatics, children can react from playing with other children who have cats or carry cat dander or saliva on them. As a result, I always clear asthmatics for cat allergen, regardless of whether or not they have their own cat.

Carol was a patient with severe asthma and eczema and severe animal, especially cat, sensitivities. In her work environment, she would react dramatically to the cat dander carried on the clothes of coworkers who had cats. It was the only allergen she could imagine that would cause such severe reactions. Her itching, pain, and wheezing were so bad that they almost disabled her. Once we had cleared her of her sensitivity to cats and dogs, to her amazement, she became allergy and symptom free. Her debilitating reactions to cat dander on her coworkers and in her workplace are completely gone.

POLLENS

Pollens, another group of inhalants, may have a more widespread effect than we previously suspected. For example, I have successfully cleared sensitivities to fruit by treating for the fruit tree pollen. And the reverse is also true; clearing for fruit and sugars can often cure sensitivities to the pollen.

Pollens cannot be avoided, but the amounts vary throughout the year. Tree pollens cause problems in the early spring, grass pollens strike in late spring and early summer, and weed pollens cause flare-ups in late summer. Seasonal patterns vary in different regions of the United States, and it is important to know the pattern in your area. For example, ragweed is at its highest level in the East Coast and Midwest regions from mid-August to late October. In temperate climates such as California, pollens are present year-round. Weather and time of day also have an effect on asthma symptoms; ragweed, for example, releases pollen in the early morning.

Ragweed is a common offender. It has been estimated that up to 75 percent of seasonal hay fever in the eastern United States is caused by ragweed. There are seventeen different species, and each plant produces up to one billion pollen grains that can be carried five hundred miles by the wind.

Pollen is produced by weeds, shrubs, grasses, flowers, and trees. When treating an asthmatic, I consider all these possibilities. I remember treating one little boy who wheezed whenever he went out to play. We cleared for flowers, weeds, and shrubs, with some improvement, but clearing him for grasses made all the difference. We recheck periodically, because new kinds of grass pollens can show up and cause problems.

SMOKE AND CHEMICALS

Other harmful inhalants include smoke, smog, pollutants, chalk, perfumes, carpet pad fumes, and formaldehyde, which is almost certainly a trigger for asthmatics. Formaldehyde is found in new clothes, clothing labels, rugs, polyurethane foam, perfumes, refinishing materials, plywood, particleboard, countertops, electronic equipment, deodorants, chlorine, and certain foods. Outdoors, its primary source is the combustion of gasoline and diesel fuel; indoors, primary sources are cigarette smoke, carpets, and furniture. Toxic pollutants can be given off by any number of building products, including wood glue, paint (acrylic, latex, and oil), paint thinner, turpentine, and pine turpines. Household products that emit fumes include chlorine bleach and other laundry products and heating fuels such as diesel, natural gas, propane, and butane. Freon, which is contained in air-conditioning systems and refrigerators, and hydrocarbons, which are chemical compounds released by the combustion of coal, oil, and gas, are problems for some asthmatics.

Although indoor smoke sensitivities can include both tobacco smoke and wood smoke, cigarette smoke is one of the most disagreeable and potentially dangerous indoor pollutants. It is made up of a complex mixture of gases and particles that contain a variety of chemicals, including synthetic compounds, added to the cigarette by the tobacco company. Indoor tobacco smoking substantially increases levels of carbon monoxide, formaldehyde, nitrogen dioxide, acrolein, hydrocarbons, hydrogen cyanide, and many other substances in a building's air. Indoor wood-burning stoves are usually used in cold, oxygen-poor conditions, which results in the release of large amounts of carbon monoxide and other inhaled chemicals and particles. Increased use of wood as a heating fuel has raised many concerns about indoor contamination. Wood smoke can be dreadful for an asthma sufferer.

SYNTHETIC FIBERS

Synthetic fiber bedding is also a source of inhalant allergens. One researcher noted: "British researchers compared 486 children who had suffered wheezing attacks in the past year to a similar sized group of healthy children. They found that children who used feather pillows were actually less likely to suffer from wheezing than those who sleep with synthetic bedding. If this is true, synthetic fiber pillows may be an important newly identified cause of severe childhood asthma and could account for half of the asthma cases seen in this study."[9]

So, although feather pillows are a wonderful nesting place for house dust mites, it may not be advisable to replace them with synthetic fiber pillows. It is possible that problems with synthetic fibers are caused by a low level release of gases. (Synthetic fibers are generally made of plastics, like polyester derived from petroleum, which may tend to release irritating organic compounds for a long period of time.) Many asthmatics who come to me have as many problems with their synthetic fiber pillows as with feather pillows. Therefore, I test them for both types of pillows and recommend that they use the kind of pillow they do not react to or that they get cleared with BioSET for one or both kinds.

Indoor Environmental Allergens

Certain allergies only occur indoors, and some asthmatics only have symptoms in their homes. Indoor environmental allergens may be the culprits.

Indoor pollution is a serious problem, with at least five hundred harmful chemicals reported in many buildings. This pollution can come from fumes from room dividers, telephone cables, paint, and carpeting. The worst offender is formaldehyde, a chemical that we discussed in the inhalant section. Some sensitive individuals react as soon as they walk into a department store because of the formaldehyde found in new clothing.

Volatile organic compounds (VOCs) are found in many household products, including dry-cleaned clothing, paint solvents, cleaning products, wood preservatives, aerosol sprays, air fresheners, stored fuels, hobby supplies, disinfectants, repellents, and automotive products. Some chemicals appear to penetrate the nasal membrane and cause congestion, runny nose, tearing eyes, and, in asthmatics, wheezing and coughing.

Asbestos is a major health hazard that was used from 1945 to 1975 in ceiling materials, synthetic tiles, acoustical wall coating, stove guards, and as insulation on hot water heaters. It is a major trigger for asthmatics.

Indoor chemical sensitivities are becoming more prevalent because there is less ventilation in tight, energy-efficient houses and buildings. Media attention has led to increased public awareness of this problem in recent years. Poor indoor air quality in buildings has been associated with a variety of syndromes or groups of symptoms loosely known as "building-related illness" or "sick-building syndrome." These terms are applied when one or more occupants in a building develop certain recognized symptoms that are apparently related to some indoor pollutant. Many of these illnesses involve hypersensitivity of the lungs and respiratory system. In one illness, called hypersensitivity pneumonitis, organic dust can create complex immune system reactions and symptoms, including mucous membrane irritation, coughing, chest tightness, headache, and fatigue. People with these illnesses are diagnosed as having multiple chemical sensitivities (MCS) or environmental illness (EI).

Chemical sensitivities can be triggered through the use of or exposure to cosmetics, perfumes, hair spray, hair products, chlorine and other cleaning products, and detergents. A common offender is dichlorobenzene, found in moth balls, insect spray, disinfectants, and solvents. A Hong Kong study suggests that poorly ventilated gas stoves may increase kids' asthma and other breathing difficulties and are likely to cause wheezing, breathlessness, and hay fever—and asthma.[10] Your car can also be filled with pollutants, from plastics, carpets, and leather preservatives. I remember a woman who had improved in her treatment until she bought a new Jeep. She had to spend a lot of time in her car for her job, and she started to cough and wheeze. When she found a small bottle of leather preservative that had been left in the glove compartment, we cleared her for it with BioSET. Since then, she has been able to drive long distances without any problem.

The house and car are not the only hazardous areas—more than half a million Americans suffer from asthma caused by breathing some kind of irritant at work. One article reported that 5–15 percent of all asthma cases are caused by on-the-job irritants.[11] These irritants can cause problems ranging from shortness of breath, wheezing, and lung inflammation to life-threatening attacks. According to the author, the most common asthma-inducing agents on the job are isocyanates, chemicals used in the manufacture of foam for chairs and car seats and in spray paint and glue. A recent report of a twelve-member panel of the American College of Chest Physicians estimates that 5 percent of workers exposed to isocyanates will develop asthma.[12] Other common workplace irritants known to cause asthma are latex, molds, animal dander, grain dust, and wood dust.

Outdoor Environmental Allergens

Environmental sensitivities resulting from outdoor pollutants, chemicals, and toxins are compromising our immune systems and causing severe health problems, especially among asthmatics.

Outdoor pollution may result from natural causes—such as the eruption of volcanoes, dust storms, or forest fires—or from human-made causes, including vehicle exhaust, fossil fuel combustion, and petroleum refining. General air pollution and smog affects us all. Many people have only burning eyes or a little congestion, but asthmatics experience difficulty breathing. There is substantial scientific evidence linking specific air pollutants to an increase in illnesses and a decrease in pulmonary function, especially in children. Sulfur dioxide can cause bronchial spasms, hives, gastrointestinal disorders, inflammation of the walls of the blood vessels (vasculitis), and related disorders. Temporary or perhaps permanent bronchial hypersensitivity has been connected to inhaling ozone, and long-term exposure to nitrogen dioxide has been associated with the increased occurrence of respiratory illness.

ARTIFICIAL TOXINS

Since the Clean Air Act went into effect in the fall of 1995, methyl tertiary-butyl ether (MTBE) has been added to gasoline to reduce the amount of carbon monoxide emissions. Unfortunately, this fuel additive is responsible for increased bronchial and lung problems, as well as skin rashes and symptoms of disorientation. Since 1999 in California and other locations, MTBE has begun to be phased out because of groundwater contamination citing unproven health effects. Most refiners have chosen to use MTBE over other oxygenates primarily for its blending characteristics and for economic reasons. It is produced from natural gas, which is cheaper than oil. In 1995 high levels of MTBE were discovered by chance in the water wells of Santa Monica, California. Subsequent U.S. findings indicate tens of thousands of contaminated sites in water wells distributed across the country. The International Agency for Research on Cancer (IARC), a World Health Organization agency, maintains that MTBE is not classifiable as a human carcinogen. However, exposure to high levels of MTBE has significant non-cancer-related health risks. Although there have not been any studies directly related to asthma, there are some anecdotal cases recorded that seem to be related to MTBE.[13]

The propellants used in metered-dose inhalants for asthmatics contain chlorofluorocarbons (CFCs), chemical agents that, when released into the air, become part of the chemical brew that can damage the Earth's ozone layer. These CFCs are also found in air-conditioning, hair sprays, cleaning solvents, and other propelled products.

Other atmospheric environmental pollutants include car exhaust, gas and diesel fuel exhaust, acid nitricom and acid sulfurosum (sulfurous acid from coal-fired plants and gasoline exhaust), and asbestos dust generated from automotive brakes in sufficient quantities to be measurable. Fumes, exhaust gases, and pesticides contain ethylene oxide; car exhaust contains cadmium sulfuricum and chromium oxydatum, a by-product of burning jet fuels; and paint (latex, oil, and so on) contains plumbum metallicum, a lead. Fertilizers sometimes contain calcium cyanimide (calcium nitrate), which is also found in foods; potassium nitrate (saltpeter); superphosphate; and thomasmeal.

NATURAL TOXINS

Radon is a naturally occurring environmental toxin, the by-product of uranium 238. It is formed in soil and rock and can accumulate in enclosed places. Risks to individuals are evaluated according to the intensity of the radiation and the length of a person's exposure to the toxin. Radon absorption occurs through inhalation and drinking groundwater. Levels are highest during the warm months of the year and are higher in lower parts of an enclosed space. There is an increased incidence of lung cancer among miners working in a high radon environment and among members of residential households with excessive levels of radon.

Many people are also sensitive to naturally occurring radiation. For example, I used to get a bad headache every time I spent time in the sun, even if I wore a hat or other head covering. Since I have been cleared for a sensitivity to radiation, I have had no problem with the sun. Natural radiation levels fluctuate and are highest during changes in weather. Some people feel sick whenever it starts to rain or the weather changes in some other way. Asthmatics especially tend to be worse during a change of weather, but treating for radiation with BioSET can change this.

Carbon dioxide may also cause a sensitivity reaction in some individuals, leading to a buildup of the gas in the bodily fluids. This sensitivity is especially apparent when people climb to higher altitudes or land or take off in an airplane, but it can also be provoked by drinking carbonated water. I have seen people suffer both asthma symptoms and migraines as a result of this allergy. In order to attain normality of the respiratory gases, people have to breathe more forcefully, which can lead to dyspnea, a mental anxiety associated with the inability to breathe enough to satisfy the demand for air. The allergy reaction to carbon dioxide is also referred to as "air hunger," an experience that most asthmatics find very frightening. Since many asthmatics are also allergic to adrenaline, this fear may make the symptoms even worse as adrenaline levels rise.

ATMOSPHERIC CHANGES

Atmospheric changes can have dramatic effects on asthmatics, especially when the temperature falls and the humidity increases. Even jumping into cold water, eating something cold, or inhaling cold air can provoke an attack. One asthmatic patient who often traveled to New York told me that as soon as she hit the cold winter weather, she would start coughing. Once we cleared her for cold, the weather no longer bothered her, and she could spend part of the year there without getting sick.

INSECT STINGS

Stinging insects include the bee, the yellow jacket, the wasp, and two types of hornets—yellow and white-faced. All of these can cause sensitivity reactions. There are six basic types of reactions to insect stings:

+ A small local reaction
+ A large local reaction
+ Urticaria, or hives, which is not life threatening
+ A life-threatening reaction, such as a swollen throat that blocks breathing
+ An asthma attack
+ Dizziness and fainting

When the throat closes off, a venom amino therapy injection, containing actual venom, may be necessary. Such injections are successful 80–100 percent of the time.

The best way to deal with stinging insects is to avoid them and take precautions: wear shoes when walking through grass; do not stand around trash receptacles; and limit the use of perfumes and avoid wearing bright colored clothing (which might attract the insects) in areas around the insects.

BioSET practitioners have had wonderful results clearing mild insect sensitivities. Once patients have been cleared, they should react less severely to being stung by that insect.

One young girl was brought in by her mother because she had apparently been stung by a bee. She had a rash, her arm was swelling, and she was in a great deal of pain. We found that she had, in fact, been stung by a wasp, and we cleared her for that sensitivity. Before she left the office, all symptoms of the sting, including the rash, had completely disappeared. I have witnessed similar results with bites from mosquitoes, bees, spiders, and ticks.

One woman patient who had been bitten by a tick brought the creature with her when she came to be treated for a reaction to the bite. By the time she left the office, all reactions to the bite were gone.

Metabolic Causes of Asthma

Metabolic causes of asthma include food sensitivities, digestive stress, and deficiencies in vitamins and minerals. The strength of our immune and respiratory systems depends on good nutrition. Reduction of food sensitivities, adequate utilization of vitamins and minerals, and reduction of digestive stress enable one to maintain a good immune response.

Food Sensitivities

Food sensitivities are a primary sensitivity for all asthmatics.

SUGARS AND CARBOHYDRATES

Carbohydrates and sugars consist of fructose, found in fruit; lactose, found in dairy products; glucose; and maltose, found in grains, pasta, breads, cereals, and vegetables. People generally eat too many carbohydrates, and carbohydrate intolerance—that is, the inability to digest sugars and starches—is quite common. Undiagnosed sugar intolerance plays a role in many kinds of sensitivities. In my practice, I routinely see sugar intolerance in patients with asthma and sinusitis. For an asthmatic or anyone with sensitivities or an immune system under stress, sugar can produce excessive amounts of mucus and can lead to severe asthmatic symptoms. Sugar sensitivities are a common cause of mucus buildup in the bronchus, the lungs, the throat, and the sinuses.

I have often seen children's immune systems severely compromised by excessive amounts of carbohydrates and sugar. These children burn themselves out more quickly than other children, their energy fades during a particular time of the day, they lack prolonged focus and attention, and they constantly crave carbohydrates and sugar. With children who come in with a chronic cough, removing sugar from their diets stops much of the coughing right away. Treating them with BioSET for a sensitivity to sugar diminishes both the craving and the cough.

Sugar is also one of the primary foods that are related to infectants, especially bacteria and fungi. Eating excessive amounts of sugar can cause a related dormant or hidden infectant to surface, beginning a cycle of infections such as ear, sinus, or bronchial infections. In children, this can result in repeated school absences.

It is also important to clear and desensitize sensitivities to protein. Many individuals are sensitive to amino acids. People who are sensitive to one or all of the amino acids do not absorb or digest them properly and cannot utilize them. This can result in a craving for protein and sugar because the body is not able to absorb sugar without the necessary amino acids. Also, 50 percent of our protein is converted to sugars, which is another reason that a sensitivity to amino acids may increase sugar craving. Since the brain requires a constant supply of glucose, it is important to check for and clear sensitivities to amino acids and proteins as well as to sugars.

When large amounts of sugars are eaten, B vitamins and minerals, especially potassium, are depleted. People who have sensitivities to B vitamins may be deficient in these vitamins because their bodies are unable to absorb and utilize them. For these people, it is important to clear the B vitamin sensitivity with BioSET before the sugar sensitivity is cleared. Otherwise, their already-low levels of B vitamins may be further depleted. B vitamin deficiency can cause depression, mental fatigue, low energy, and exhaustion.

Sugar is also responsible for bloating in many people, and it is strongly linked to fungi infections. I have found that people who are sensitive to B vitamins and sugar are especially likely to have fungi infections.

A craving for carbohydrates and sugars is always a result of B vitamin problems. When people tell me that they crave complex carbohydrates, I always look for B vitamin and sugar sensitivities. When people crave sugars, I look for the amino acid as well as the B vitamin sensitivities.

FATS

Fats need to be digested well in order for the body to utilize the fatty acids necessary for the nervous system's health. Fatty acids help to control neurotransmitters and assist in the manufacture and secretion of vital hormones in the thyroid, adrenal, and pituitary glands. They also act as antioxidants and inhibit the secretion of acid in the stomach. Clearing sensitivities to fats can be very beneficial to asthmatics.

DAIRY PRODUCTS

A sensitivity to dairy products such as milk, yogurt, and cheese is one of the most common and widely recognized forms of food sensitivities. I have found that dairy product sensitivities can often be eliminated by clearing sensitivities to calcium, casein, albumin, and the sugar lactose. Sometimes the specific dairy product itself needs to be cleared. With the full BioSET treatment, including enzymes, a dairy intolerance or sensitivity can be reduced.

One of the most common complaints with dairy product sensitivity is excess mucus. Probably all of us have had this experience at some time or another—the need to clear our throats after eating a certain food. I remember one woman who constantly had mucus in her throat, especially after she ate dairy products. After we cleared her with BioSET, she no longer had the problem with any food, including dairy. She was surprised because, being in the health field, she believed that dairy products are always mucus producing. Before working with this method, I had held the same idea and was equally surprised by our results.

EGGS

Since so many people are extremely sensitive to eggs, this food can certainly be a trigger for asthma. Eggs can often be cleared simply by clearing amino acids early in the BioSET treatment protocol.

SOY PRODUCTS

The soybean is a vegetarian source of protein, but it is also frequently a sensitivity. Many mothers tell me they take their children off milk early and put them on rice and soy milks. The mothers mean well, but this practice may result in children with chronic upper respiratory infections that are caused by their sensitivity to soy.

Soy is now being used to make milk, cheese, nuts, flour, and vegetarian "meat," with new products coming out all the time. Lecithin is a soy product that is often used in candy to prevent drying and to help emulsify the fats. For this reason, clearing lecithin can often clear a chocolate sensitivity. Soy is also used in many other foods where you might not expect it. Soy flour is used in hard candies, fudge, nut candies, and caramels. Some bakeries use soy milk instead of cow's milk. Soy products are used in custards and in coffee substitutes, as well as in household products such as varnish, paints, enamels, printing ink, massage creams, celluloid, paper finishes, cloth, nitro-glycerin, some dog food, adhesives, soap, fertilizer, automobile parts, textiles, and lubricating oil. As soy becomes more common in the environment, it is important that sensitive people be treated for it.

GRAINS

Corn is a major grain sensitivity. Many foods you might not expect to contain corn do so in the form of cornstarch or corn syrup. Most prepared foods contain cornstarch, as does Chinese food, baking powder, and toothpaste. It is the binding product in most pills and vitamins, including aspirin, Tylenol, and other kinds of drugs. Corn syrup is a common sweetener found in many soft drinks. Corn is also often found in food mixes, canned foods, and foods cooked in corn oil. And corn silk is used in many makeup products.

Another common grain to which people are sensitive is wheat. Foods that contain wheat are so numerous that I have listed them in appendix A.

Barley, oats, and rye can also be sensitivities. BioSET practitioners generally advocate a no-grain diet for most everyone, especially asthmatics. Sugars and grains contribute to a multitude of health problems for which people routinely resort to medications for relief. Asthmatics and sinus sufferers experience a complete health turnaround once they wean themselves from sugars and grains. Thus we advise our patients to steer clear of sugars, grains, and the foods that contain them, including cookies, candies, crackers, breads, cereals, pastas, and even energy bars, which contain large amounts of carbohydrates. Instead, build your diet around vegetables and especially fruits, and proteins such as fish, poultry, beans, nuts, and oils.[1] You may ask, why don't we just clear for grains, and then allow people to eat them even if just on a limited basis? Based on experience, I have found that grains cannot be cleared due to metabolic components commonly referred to as anti-nutrients. Anti-nutrients can provoke an autoimmune response, an aggressive response during which the body attacks its own tissues. Eliminating grains is the only option, and for asthmatics, this is profound. The change in their symptoms when avoiding all grains can be overwhelming. This holds true for those with asthma and sinusitis as well as with autoimmune disorders.

FRUITS

Any fruit can be a potential allergen. I have seen people sensitive to just about all of them, including apples, bananas, grapes, pears, melons, the more acid fruits such as pineapples, strawberries, and kiwi, and the more sugary fruits such as papaya and mangoes. Many children drink too much apple juice, which can be mucus forming. Both apple juice and bananas can in particular create problems for asthmatics. The chemicals that are sprayed on fruit can also be a problem and can be serious triggers for asthmatics.

Treating for vitamin C and sugars can often clear these fruit allergies, as can clearing for common ingredients in fruits such as acid, phenolics (which give food its color, flavor, and odor), and salicylates (which function as preservatives).

PEANUTS

Peanuts are a widely used food and a common food allergen and sensitivity. The incidence of peanut allergy and/or sensitivity has increased in the last decade, perhaps because of the increased use of peanut products and of peanut butter as a source of protein. Research has indicated that many lactating mothers use peanut butter to supplement their protein intake while breastfeeding. Because peanut allergen is secreted in breast milk, this can create a sensitivity in an at-risk child.

Reactions from peanuts can include mucus formation, asthmatic attacks, and, for those who are allergic, anaphylactic shock. BioSET practitioners can clear adults and children successfully for peanut sensitivity unless there is an IgE immune reaction to peanuts, which can be very severe and is beyond the scope of the BioSET practice. Other nuts to which people are often sensitive are cashews, pecans, and walnuts.

NIGHTSHADES

Eggplants, potatoes, tomatoes, and peppers are all members of the nightshade family. Any of them can be serious sensitivities and can provoke immediate asthmatic reactions. I have also seen the nightshades act as irritants for arthritics or others with joint pain. Sometimes what is diagnosed as arthritis is actually a sensitivity to one of these foods. Studies have indicated that a sensitivity to eggplant is linked to certain grass and other allergies, such as ragweed, birch, or animal dander.

VEGETABLES

Many vegetables are potential sensitivities. Onions are known to be a common trigger for asthmatics. Peppers and potatoes are sometimes a problem (see the section on nightshades), as are yams, cucumbers, and carrots. Carrots can be a powerful allergen; in fact, I have seen people begin wheezing immediately after eating a carrot. Sometimes clearing for vitamin A or other phenolics (ingredients found in or added to foods that give them their flavor, color, and odor, to which some people are sensitive) will clear a sensitivity to carrots, without having to clear for the carrots themselves. For example, before being cleared for vitamin A, I used to suffer a dull headache and nausea after eating carrots, but not anymore. Dried beans can also be a problem, especially garbanzo, kidney, and pinto beans.

FISH, SEAFOOD, AND MEAT

Fish and seafood can cause severe asthmatic reactions. Turkey, chicken, and pheasant are also common sensitivities. In fact, I have found chicken to be the most common food allergen. A turkey sensitivity is sometimes a reaction to the amino acid tryptophan in turkey, which is the precursor to the neurotransmitter serotonin (in other words, tryptophan can be made into serotonin). A tryptophan sensitivity, which may implicate serotonin, can produce feelings of depression, tiredness, and mental fogginess.

CHOCOLATE, CAFFEINE, AND COFFEE

People commonly have sensitivities to chocolate and caffeine. In fact, a craving for chocolate usually indicates a sensitivity to it. In addition to obvious sources such as coffee and tea, caffeine is also a hidden ingredient in some soft drinks and over-the-counter medications such as Excedrin and other aspirin-based products. Both the sensitivity to caffeine and the sensitivity to chocolate, which tend to result in heavy mucous production and congestion, can be treated with BioSET.

I had one patient who ate excessive amounts of chocolate her whole life and noticed that she coughed after eating it. Once, as we were clearing her for something else, she ate some chocolate and began to cough deeply and wheeze, like an asthmatic. When I cleared her for the chocolate, the coughing stopped immediately. Her craving disappeared, and she never again coughed after eating it.

SALT AND SPICES

Surprisingly, common table salt has been indicated as an asthma trigger. A recent study suggests a correlation between levels of salt intake and asthma symptoms, especially among men. High salt intake is also correlated with deaths from asthma in men and children. Other studies have shown increased bronchial activity in men with high salt intake, but not in women.[2]

Most asthmatics have sensitivities to spices. For example, garlic is a common allergen, though regarded by many as a healthy food. I have seen asthmatics who began wheezing after eating excessive amounts of garlic. It can also cause indigestion, bloating, and headaches. Vanilla and artificial sweeteners are allergens to some people.

MINERALS

Minerals such as iodine, lead, magnesium, manganese, zinc, sulfur, silver, and vanadium can also be a problem for some individuals.

FLUORIDE

Fluoride, another asthma trigger, is found naturally in certain foods and is added to the water supply in many areas. Recent studies show an increase of certain chronic health problems with exposure to fluoride.[3] Though much has been written about the benefits of fluoride, people need to educate themselves about the possible dangers as well.

Food Additives

Many common food additives can cause problems for asthmatics and other sensitive people. These include sulfites, MSG, hydrolyzed vegetable protein, sodium nitrate, and sodium nitrite. Sulfites in particular are potentially deadly for asthmatics. I have seen several cases of children who had serious reactions after eating in fast food restaurants. Most food additives are listed on prepared foods, but the law does not require that small amounts be mentioned, so sensitive people might eat them without being aware of it. Preservatives like BHA and BHT, which are used in packaging, also may cause reactions in sensitive people who eat the food contained in that packaging.

MSG (monosodium glutamate) has been used for many years as a flavor enhancer for a variety of foods prepared at home and in restaurants. Manufactured by a fermentation process using starch, beet sugar, and cane sugar or molasses, MSG is the sodium salt of glutamic acid, an amino acid that is found naturally in our bodies. Glutamic acid makes up a large part of the proteins found in foods such as cheese, meat, peas, mushrooms, and milk.

The FDA has studied many of the reportedly adverse effects of MSG but, unfortunately, still considers it a safe ingredient. BioSET practitioners disagree because we have cleared many people who are sensitive to MSG and find that it causes particular problems for asthmatics.

Any packaged food that contains MSG must list this ingredient on the label. Other food ingredients that contain glutamate include hydrolyzed vegetable proteins, autolyzed yeast, extract flavorings, natural flavorings, and potassium glutamate. Hydrolyzed vegetable protein contains 5–20 percent glutamate and is used in place of MSG as a flavor enhancer in many foods such as canned tuna, dried soup mixes, canned vegetables, and processed meats. People who are sensitive to MSG may be sensitive to other glutamate products as well. Be aware that MSG and the other glutamates do not have to be listed as ingredients if they are a component of an ingredient that is listed, such as hydrolyzed vegetable protein. This can have serious consequences for people who are sensitive and have no way of knowing that they are eating these additives.

It is important to check labels in any case. Look for MSG in dips, soup mixes, stews, gravy, sauces, prepared meats, poultry, fish, and vegetables. In restaurants that claim they do not use MSG, you might still get MSG in the commercial sauces or spice mixes used since restaurant owners do not realize these foods contain one of the glutamates. Since it is difficult to avoid MSG and the other glutamates completely, it is best to be cleared for them if you are sensitive. I have had excellent results in clearing for sensitivities to MSG, hydrolyzed vegetable proteins and other glutamates, and other food additives. If you are not sensitive to them, your body will be able to eliminate them quickly and easily.

Gums, such as acacia, karaya, xanthum, and tragacanth gums, are another kind of additive that can cause problems. They are found in many foods, including yogurt, candy bars, cottage cheese, soft drinks, soy sauce, barbecue sauce, macaroni and cheese, and ready-made foods.

Some other additives include acidum ascorbicum, the sorbic acid found in canned meats; acidum benzoicum, a food preservative; dipthenyl, a preservative for oranges; and hexamethylenetetramine, a preservative used in canned fruit. Sodium pyrophosphoricum gives the red color to meat, especially processed meats. Sodium phenol phenolate, sodium sulfurosum, sorbic acid, and urethanum, which are used in wine manufacturing, and carbamide, which is used to inhibit potato sprouting, may all produce reactions.

Another major additive group is the salicylates, food preservatives that are used, among other places, in the manufacture of aspirin. Many asthmatics have problems with salicylate foods, though they appear to build up in the system before provoking a reaction.

Salicylate is both a food additive and a substance that appears naturally in many foods. Salicylate food may be tolerated on a four-day rotation diet, but not if eaten every day. Most sensitive individuals will not react every time the food is eaten, unless it is consumed in excessive amounts. Salicylates are found in a variety of fruits, including apples, apricots, blackberries, boysenberries, cantaloupe, cherries, cranberries, dates, guava, grapes, loganberries, oranges, pineapples, plums, dark red raspberries, frozen strawberries, gooseberries, and currants. They are also found in vegetables such as chicory, chili peppers, endive, mushrooms, sweet and green peppers, radishes, tomato paste, tomato sauce, zucchini, almonds, peanuts, water chestnuts, bay leaves, basil, caraway, champagne, chili flakes, chili powder, ginger root, mint, nutmeg, cloves, green olives, white pepper, peppermint, port, tea bags, herbal teas, vanilla flavoring, and wine vinegar. A variety of crackers, some cereals, cake mixes, muffins, biscuits, cakes, coffee, pastries, tobacco, mayonnaise, ketchup, Jell-O and gelatin, candies, gum, and corned beef contain them as well.

Food coloring is another important category of additives. I discuss some case histories involving food coloring in a later section. Many candies, like jelly beans, contain large amounts of coloring. Even foods sold in natural food stores may contain coloring, so beware. Reactions to food coloring can be serious, from a severe constriction of air passageways to coughing, runny nose, and fever.

PESTICIDES

Though many people do not think of them as such, pesticides can be thought of as food additives, and they are particularly serious because they are everywhere. Even banned pesticides such as DDT still exist in residues in the soil and in people's bodies. I have tested several people who register a sensitivity to DDT. I remember treating one man who was HIV positive and suffered from severe fatigue and a depressed immune system. One of the breakthroughs in our treatment occurred when I cleared him for pesticides, to which he was highly allergic. He told me that he grew up on a farm and had helped his father spray the plants and trees with pesticides.

Of course, ideally people should eat organic foods that are free of pesticides, but pesticides are so pervasive in the environment that they are very difficult to avoid. For this reason, BioSET practitioners often clear patients for sensitivities to them.

ALCOHOL

Beer, wine, and liquor cause difficulties for many people, and the alcoholic content of these beverages is the root of the problem. BioSET practitioners first clear for B vitamins and sugars, then for alcohol. In fact, our clinic has successfully cleared several alcoholics of their addiction to alcohol, and, with the help of other therapies, they have successfully recovered. Often the craving for alcohol is a craving for sugar and the B vitamins that have been depleted by alcohol consumption. Of course, it is a vicious circle, because drinking alcohol further depletes many B vitamins and minerals.

Alcohol is not just a problem for those who drink alcoholic beverages. Anyone who consumes large amounts of fruits and sugars will naturally produce alcohol. For myself, alcohol was a difficult sensitivity to clear. Although I did not drink it often, I ate lots of fruit, and I was showing signs of becoming addicted. After I was cleared for alcohol and sugars, my cravings diminished. From that point on I also noticed that when I did drink alcohol, I no longer had headaches, depression, or the other symptoms I formerly experienced.

Alcoholic beverages made from grains will cause a negative reaction for anyone sensitive to these grains. Alcohol also tends to aggravate or sustain yeast and other fungus infections. Since beer and wine are made with yeast, they will cause problems for anyone with fungal sensitivities. Therefore, it is important to eliminate alcohol cravings when clearing for fungi, especially with asthmatics, who tend to have a problem with excessive fungi. Both the yeast and alcohol in beer may cause difficulties. Wines contain other ingredients that can be problematic as well—sulfites, which I discussed, and histamines, which I will talk about in the next chapter.

WATER

Surprisingly enough, some people react to their drinking water. One woman told me that she thought she was sensitive to the bottled spring water she used. Every time she drank it, she coughed. When I tested her, I found that she was indeed sensitive. When she stopped drinking the water, her cough went away and her mucous production diminished significantly. People who are sensitive to bottled water may be reacting to something in the water, such as fluoride or some minerals, or to the plastic containers in which the water is bottled. Some people even seem to be sensitive to their tap water.

PHENOLICS

Phenolics are derivatives of benzene that are used to give flavor and color to foods, and to help preserve them. They also occur naturally in some foods. Once phenolics enter the bloodstream, they are broken down in the liver and excreted into the intestines in bile or eliminated in the urine. Cow's milk naturally contains high levels of phenolics and will often provoke a reaction. Since there are *fourteen different* phenolics in milk, people cleared for cow's milk, which might normally desensitize them, may continue to react to phenolics until specifically cleared for them. Tomatoes, soybeans, and soybean products are also high in phenolics.

Some of the phenolics that asthmatics react to most often are cinnamic acid, coumarin, dopamine, gallic acid, histamine, indole, malvin, phenylisothiocyanate, rutin, and uric acid.

Cinnamic acid is found most often in fruits, tomatoes, cheese, lettuce, bananas, and such juices as apple, grape, orange, pineapple, and tomato. Coumarin is found in about thirty different foods, the most common being wheat, rice, barley, corn, soy, cheese, beef, and eggs. Coumarin has been used commercially as a flavor for tobacco, butter, and medicines. When someone has a wheat allergy, it may be because of the coumarin, so it is important to test and clear for wheat and for all of the phenolics.

Dopamine is a neurotransmitter involved with inhibition, coordination, and integration of fine muscular movement, such as picking up small objects. It is also involved with memory and emotions. Dopamine has been shown to play a role in Parkinson's disease and has been linked with high copper levels in schizophrenics. There are high levels of dopamine in pineapples, bananas, plantain, and avocados.

Gallic acid, found in some 70 percent of all foods, including food-coloring agents, is unquestionably one of the two most common phenolics, along with coumarin. It can act as an asthmatic trigger; cause chronic nasal congestion, sinusitis, and chronic fatigue; and lead to hyperactivity in children.

Histamine is an immune mediator that can cause many allergic responses in response to sensitivities. Symptoms such as congestion, difficulty breathing, and red eyes are all common reactions to histamine sensitivities.

Bacteria break down the amino acid tryptophan to form indole and skatole. When indole is detectable in feces, it indicates bowel toxicity and fermentation of food by putrefactive bacteria. Indole is found in all complete proteins. When ingested, it penetrates the gut and moves into the liver, where it is converted into alcohol and excreted in the urine. Excessive production of indole can be carcinogenic. It is found in oranges, flowers, green vegetables, and, in high levels, in dairy products. It is also found in perfumes. When BioSET practitioners find high levels of indole in laboratory tests and a person is suffering from bloating and constipation, we suspect poor protein digestion. Based on indole levels and other markers, we will recommend enzymes to help digest protein. Chronic bowel problems are fairly common among asthmatics, but they can be cleared for indole, skatole, and other byproducts of bowel elimination.

Malvin, found in more than thirty foods, is the natural red and blue pigment in fruits and vegetables such as strawberries, tomatoes, and Concord grapes. It is also found in oranges, eggs, chicken, milk, soy foods, vegetables, and dairy products. Like gallic acid and coumarin, it is a common cause of reactions.

Phenylisothiocyanate is found in twenty foods, including chicken, eggs, beets, soybeans, cheese, lamb, peanuts, and legumes. This phenolic can stimulate the sympathetic nervous system and may be a cause of migraines.

Rutin, a bioflavonoid containing glucose and quercetin, is found in about fifty foods, including eggs and rice, and in plants such as buckwheat, hydrangea, pansies, ragweed, and goldenrod. A rutin deficiency or a sensitivity to rutin can cause a susceptibility to bruising. This is such a common allergen that it is one of the first that BioSET practitioners deal with when we begin clearing treatments.

Uric acid is present in the urine of all carnivorous animals and in cat saliva. The end product of the nitrogenous metabolism of protein, it appears in the urine when the plasma concentration is slightly higher than normal. A high concentration of uric acid in the urine is an indication of poor protein metabolism or excess protein consumption. It may also be an indication of stones or calculi in the kidneys or bladder and may be linked to gout, hepatitis, and leukemia. Certain foods, including caffeine, beans, nicotine, meat, spinach, and mushrooms, can produce high uric acid levels.

BioSET practitioners have had excellent results clearing asthmatics for phenolics. Not only does this help reduce asthma symptoms, it helps desensitize people to many foods that contain phenolics.

Digestion

The by-products of poor digestion can cause sensitivity reactions. Any undigested food—whether protein, carbohydrate, fat, or fiber—can be absorbed into the bloodstream and regarded by the immune system as an allergen. In evaluating and clearing allergens in our clinic, digestion is a key factor. Having proper digestion is crucial, because without it, the clearing of sensitivities may be neither successful nor permanent. I stress optimal digestion and discuss it with everyone who comes to see me. (See my book *MicroMiracles: Discover the Healing Power of Enzymes.*)

BioSET practitioners encourage adequate chewing of food to help predigest it as well as taking a full-spectrum vegetarian digestive enzyme to guarantee complete digestion of each meal. In our experience and in our practice, we have found that digestive enzymes usually eliminate sensitivity to many foods. The foods that are not automatically cleared with enzymes can be cleared with BioSET. Enzymes can be a lifesaver for asthmatics and can prevent them from developing new sensitivities.

Little-Known Causes of Asthma

In chapters 5 and 6 I covered some of the most obvious causes of asthma. In this chapter I provide both practitioners and patients with insights into some of the less obvious causes of asthma. The findings outlined in this chapter are the results of years of clinical research by BioSET practitioners clearing patients for often-unsuspected causes of asthma.

Contactants

Contactants are allergens that affect the body through skin contact, and can be a surprisingly severe trigger for asthma.

LATEX

Latex is a common but largely unrecognized contactant. Over the past several years, latex has been used more frequently in a variety of professions. More than a hundred thousand health care workers, such as dentists, doctors, nurses, and lab technicians, are exposed to latex on the job. Latex is used in hospitals and medical practices for such items as anesthetic tubing and ventilation bags. People with high exposure to latex and a history of sensitivities are at risk for a reaction, as are people who have had frequent surgical procedures. Dermatitis and rashes may be irritated by latex exposure. Studies in the United States and Britain have found that the body produces specific antibodies to high levels of latex.

The American College of Allergy, Asthma, and Immunology (ACAAI) has called for the protection of health care workers and consumers, who are said to use over seven million metric tons of latex every year. Common consumer products made with latex include balloons, condoms, tires, waistbands, rubber toys, nipples, and pacifiers. The ACAAI has encouraged implementation of FDA regulations that require labeling latex, banning the "hypoallergenic" label on some latex gloves, and regulating maximum amounts of extractable allergen in latex products. The organization also recommends improved testing for the sensitivity, identifying nonallergenic forms of latex, creating latex "safe" zones in workplaces, and researching the cause of latex sensitivities.[1]

BioSET practitioners offer an alternative approach. We have treated many people successfully for serious latex sensitivities. Many of them were able to continue using latex in their jobs for their protection and the protection of their clients. One patient was a nurse practitioner who had to wear latex all the time, which exacerbated her asthma. Since her clearing with BioSET, she has been able to wear latex on the job without any problems. BioSET provides a way to deal with this new and growing problem.

CHEMICALS

Many other chemicals act as contact allergens, and more are found to be problems every year. The following is a list of contact chemicals used in a wide variety of cleaning, makeup, and fabric products that BioSET practitioners have found to be particularly problematic for asthmatics:

+ Acetone, in nail polish remover
+ Methanol
+ Benzyl alcohol
+ Ethylene oxide
+ Butter yellow
+ Tipa white
+ Congo red
+ Estradiol benzoate-8
+ Sulfurea
+ Carbon tetrachloride, used for dry cleaning
+ Trichloroethylene
+ Chromium oxide
+ Benzinum crudum
+ Mangan peroxydatum
+ Plumbum bromatum

- Plumbum sulfuricum
- Polyester
- Dimethyl terephthalate
- Ethylene glycol
- Isopropyl glycol, found in many cosmetics and deodorant sprays
- Polychlorinated biphenyls, found in pigments and dyes
- Laundry detergent
- Hydrazine sulfate
- Toluene
- Zylene
- Asbestos
- Benzanthracene
- Cyclohexanol
- Anylalcohol

FABRICS AND DYES

With asthmatics it is important to clear for fabrics, because any fabric, natural or synthetic, can cause a reaction. BioSET practitioners have cleared people for reactions to cotton, linen, wool, rayon, nylon, acetate, acrylic, polyester, and silk. Leather can also be a problem, particularly for those who are sensitive to animal dander or tannic acid. (A tannic acid sensitivity can also cause a reaction to tea.) BioSET practitioners have seen miraculous results from treating for fabrics. One patient's ability to smell and taste was restored. Another's long-term eczema subsided, and yet another client felt more focused and energetic. Itching, dry skin, and chronic ailments may all decrease dramatically or disappear after treatment. Clearing for the dyes in fabrics is also important in desensitizing people to clothing, wallpaper, mattresses, bedding, and towels.

I remember a parent who brought her daughter a bedsheet decorated with Disney characters. Every time the girl slept on it, she would get congested and begin to cough. I found that she was sensitive to the dyes in the fabric as well as to the fabric itself, polyester. Once she was cleared for these sensitivities, she could sleep on the sheet without any problems.

Some of the most sensitive fabric dyes to clear are

- Aniline, the blue-black dye used in newsprint
- Anthracene, used in the manufacture of most dye stuffs and fixed with formaldehyde

- ✦ Anthracinone, a commercial vat dye
- ✦ Benzene, used in dye manufacturing
- ✦ Bromine, used in organic dyes
- ✦ Chromium oxydatum, a dye used in tannin and in the ink on dollar bills

WOOD

Wood resin is another allergenic contactant. BioSET practitioners have seen people sensitive to wood, musical instruments, a violin bow, piano keys, the wood of a harp, and the finishing on wood.

DAILY CONTACTANTS

Insects of all kinds can be contactants, as can many common household products, including cosmetics, soaps, skin creams, detergents, gloves, hair dyes, gasoline, acrylic nails, nail polish and remover, metals (such as silver, nickel, and gold), jewelry, metal polishes, celluloid, and flowers and bulbs. Printers are often sensitive to a fine lacquer spray that is used for drying ink to keep it from smudging. Many people are also sensitive to computers, computer keyboards, phones, Naugahyde chairs, milk containers, and other disposable products. BioSET practitioners have found women to be sensitive to their panty hose, and other people sensitive to toilet paper and paper towels. Silicone, which is found in glass doors, breast implants, and the newest organic fabrics, also can cause sensitivity reactions in some people.

Other contactants include plant oils, such as those found in poison oak and poison ivy. Asparagus fern is a common trigger for asthmatics. Other ferns, jute, and kapok fabrics can also provoke reactions. Synthetic contactants include adhesive tape, cement, paper products, crude oil, plastics, newsprint, and photocopy paper and materials. One asthmatic would cough each time she read a magazine in my office. Sure enough, when she was tested, she was found to be sensitive to the ink. When she was cleared with BioSET, she no longer coughed when she read her papers and magazines. BioSET practitioners have also treated many people who were sensitive to the plastic or other material in their eyeglasses or contact lenses.

Histamines

Histamine is a very important sensitivity that plays a major role in all sensitivity reactions. Histamine is a primary neurotransmitter in the brain, especially in the hippocampus, and throughout the nervous system. It can stimulate the secretion of hydrochloric acid, an important digestive aid, in the stomach.

Studies indicate that about 20 percent of schizophrenics are high in histamine.[2] Rheumatoid arthritics and Parkinson's patients are low in histamine.[3]

All allergic individuals, especially asthmatics, have high levels of IgE (immunoglobulin E) antibodies. When an allergen such as dust reacts with an IgE reagent antibody, an allergen-reagent reaction takes place, and the individual experiences a sensitivity reaction. IgE antibodies attach to mast cells (immune cells located around the airways) and basophilis (similar to mast cells), causing them to rupture and release histamine. Increased levels of histamine cause blood vessels to dilate and smooth muscle cells to contract. A number of different abnormal symptoms can occur, depending on the type of tissue where the histamine is released. Asthma symptoms are one reaction. A sensitivity to histamine greatly intensifies reactions to other allergens.

Besides asthma symptoms, a sensitivity to histamine can cause depression, fatigue, hay fever, hyperactivity, hypertension, night sweats, PMS sinusitis, stomach pain, and vertigo. Histamine is found in wine, beer, oysters, perch, salmon, scallops, shrimp, trout, tuna fish, codfish, flounder, halibut, haddock, lobster, black bass, catfish, crabmeat, yeast mix, human milk, cow and goat milk, cocoa, mutton, ham, chicken, and turkey.

I always check asthmatics whose sensitivities are especially active, and those with severe eczema or skin reaction, for a sensitivity to histamine. I have found clearing for histamine to be highly successful and have seen remarkable changes in patients.

Hormones and Glands

BioSET practitioners have obtained many positive results by clearing asthma sufferers for adrenal and thyroid hormones, as well as for the glands themselves.

ADRENAL GLANDS

The adrenal glands lie above the kidneys and are composed of two parts, the adrenal medulla and the adrenal cortex. Each of these parts secretes different hormones. The adrenal medulla secretes adrenaline and norepinephrine. The adrenal cortex secretes corticosteroids, glycol corticoids, and androgens.

When tissue is damaged by trauma, infection, allergy, or in some other way, the tissue becomes inflamed. In some circumstances the inflammation is more damaging than the trauma or infection. Cortisol reduces all aspects of the inflammatory process by blocking the inflammatory response. With asthmatics, it is very important that this gland functions normally and is able to secrete cortisol in a natural form. If artificial sources such as cortisone, prednisone, methylprednisone, or dexamethasone are taken for prolonged periods to remedy a shortage of cortisol, they can suppress the immune system. This suppression causes reduced numbers of lymphocytes, T cells, and antibodies, which not only increases the incidence of sensitivities but makes a person more susceptible to infections and can cause chronic health problems later in life.

With BioSET, every sensitive individual is tested and cleared for their own adrenal hormones. Asthmatics always have positive results after this clearing. They feel more energetic, less sensitive to their surroundings, and less in need of their steroids and other drugs. If people are sensitive to their own hormones, they may not be able to properly absorb them into their tissues, and could develop a deficiency.

THYROID GLAND

The thyroid, a gland located immediately below the larynx on either side of and anterior to the trachea (windpipe), secretes the hormones thyroxin (90 percent) and triiodothyronine (10 percent). These hormones, respectively called T4 and T3, increase an individual's metabolic rate. The thyroid stimulates all aspects of carbohydrate metabolism, including rapid uptake by the cells and increased enzymatic activity, and enhances the metabolism of fats. The thyroid can influence both the heart rate and blood volume. Since most thyroxin is eventually converted to T3 in the liver and other tissues of the body, a healthy liver is essential for thyroid production and function. The thyroid also secretes calcitonin, an important hormone for calcium metabolism. When the rate of thyroid hormone production increases, most endocrine gland secretions increase as well, including the production of adrenal corticoid. In treating asthma, it is important to note that the thyroid can also increase the rate of oxygen utilization and the formation of carbon dioxide, thereby increasing the rate and depth of respiration. The thyroid has many other effects on the body as well.

Unfortunately, many people are sensitive to their own thyroid gland or thyroid hormones. Eighty to ninety percent of the women I have seen in the BioSET clinic are hypothyroid, though most are unaware of it. Symptoms include dry skin, cold hands and feet, tiredness, insomnia, eczema, overweight or underweight, sluggishness, hair loss, and poor memory.

If people are secreting enough T4, thyroxin, but are sensitive to their own hormone, they might not be utilizing it and can be just as hypothyroid as those with low thyroid function. This may also be the case if there is a problem converting T4 to T3, for example, if someone has a liver dysfunction. Those individuals will show the same symptoms of hypothyroid, yet the condition is not likely to show up in blood tests.

ESTROGEN, PROGESTERONE, AND DHEA

Some people are also sensitive to the female hormones estrogen and progesterone, the male hormone testosterone, and DHEA, which is an adrenal hormone. I have found reactions to insulin, androgen, and hormones related to the kidneys and their function.

Hormones that increase during premenstrual and menstrual periods and during pregnancy can trigger asthmatic attacks in women who are sensitive to their own hormones. If the asthma happens premenstrually, the trigger is usually progesterone. Postmenstrually, there are higher levels of estrogen, and in pregnancy there are higher levels of progesterone again.

A sensitivity to progesterone could produce symptoms such as premenstrual syndrome, breast tenderness, bloating, depression, and irritability prior to the start of a woman's period. People with estrogen sensitivities are more prone to uterine fibroids, ovarian cysts, fibrocystic breasts, painful periods, and migraines at the start and end of periods. Many women are sensitive to both hormones. Menopausal symptoms can also be brought on by a sensitivity to one or both hormones.

One patient of mine had PMS with migraines, increased asthmatic symptoms, irritability, and increased cravings for sugar and other foods. When I cleared her for progesterone, both her headaches and her asthma symptoms decreased immediately. In women, we have noticed that clearing for hormones is often effective in dealing with migraines. In men, the cause tends to be something like coffee, caffeine, or chocolate.

Treating for hormone sensitivities can be particularly effective for women who developed asthma later in life. One study found that women who had taken estrogen for ten years or more were twice as likely to develop asthma as women who had never taken the hormone.[4] Another study looked at ninety thousand women with past or current estrogen use and found that it doubled the chances of getting asthma. This means that women who are considering hormone replacement therapy should check their sensitivity to these hormones to prevent late-onset asthma.

Women also may react to thyroid hormone levels during different points on the menstrual cycle as well. Clearing for sensitivities to the thyroid and thyroid hormones is often helpful in balancing and regulating the menstrual cycle. After clearing for progesterone, I recommend natural progesterone oils (taken orally) or creams (used topically) made from yams and soybeans to increase progesterone levels. When people are sensitive to progesterone, they are usually deficient, and supplementation is often necessary.

A sensitivity to adrenal hormones can also be cleared with BioSET and treated with enzyme therapy. These hormones are important to women both premenopausally and postmenopausally. Taking the enzymes and having BioSET clearings during pregnancy are completely safe and can benefit both a woman and her child.

CLEARING FOR HORMONES

When BioSET practitioners find people sensitive to the thyroid and adrenal glands and their respective hormones, we clear them with BioSET and give them enzyme formulas, if necessary, to support glandular function. If we find a sensitivity to the thyroid, we will also treat a person for iodine, vegetable and animal fat, tyrosine and tryptophan (amino acids), the thyroid-stimulating hormones secreted by the pituitary, and the adrenal glands and adrenal hormones, especially cortisone.

Acid- and Alkaline-Forming Foods

Acidic foods are sour and contain the element hydrogen. The sour taste of oranges and lemons, for example, is due to the acid that they contain. Alkalines, or bases, have properties opposite to acids, and they neutralize acids. In our body fluids, blood, and extracellular fluids, acid and alkaline maintain a constant condition of alkalinity or acidity.

Foods can be acidic or alkaline, or they can be acid- or alkaline-forming. The first category refers to how much acid or alkaline the foods contain. The second refers to the condition the foods cause in the body after being metabolized. Protein, for example, is an acid-forming food because acid is the by-product of its metabolism. The same is true of grains. Fruits and most vegetables oxidize when broken down and are considered alkaline-forming foods. The following lists some common acid- and alkaline-forming foods:

Acid-Forming

Eggs	Sugar
Grains	Nuts
Meat	Beans
Fish	

Alkaline-Forming

Salt	Fruit
Vegetables	Wine

Moderate, severe, and childhood asthma sufferers are commonly sensitive to acid-forming foods, and they tend to become more metabolically acidic (acidosis) after eating them. This acidity can cause sluggishness and an increased rate and depth of respiration, which can trigger an asthmatic attack. Excessive acidity can also cause gastritis, or reflux, which can irritate the mucous membranes of the stomach, duodenum, or esophagus—a condition commonly known as heartburn. This condition can even be the precursor to an ulcer.

One authority estimates that over 75 percent of the millions of asthmatics in the United States suffer from the kind of heartburn known as gastric reflux, where stomach acid backs up into the esophagus, causing a burning sensation.[5] Since acid in the airways could increase the incidence of asthmatic reactions, he suggests testing for acid levels by using a probe in the throat and stomach to measure acid levels for twenty-four hours. If high acid levels are found, he recommends treatment with prescription drugs or surgery.

BioSET practitioners use much less invasive techniques because we believe the reflux reaction may be due to a sensitivity to foods high in acids. Sugars, which are major allergens for asthmatics, are high in acid. Acid in the airways may provoke an intense sensitivity reaction in that tissue. A sensitivity can be detected and cleared with BioSET. A gastric antacid enzyme taken at night is also very helpful. (See chapter 13 for more information on enzyme therapy.)

Vitamins and Minerals

Vitamins are important supplements for asthmatics, but many people are sensitive to the vitamins they need to take. People tend to be deficient in the vitamins to which they are sensitive because their bodies are unable to absorb and utilize them. Asthmatics are most commonly sensitive to vitamin C, all the B vitamins, vitamin A, and vitamin F, or fatty acids.

VITAMIN C

We all know that vitamin C has a wide range of applications in treating and preventing many diseases. Studies have shown it to be important to immune system health, and many books have been written about its benefits and the effects of deficiencies. It is necessary for healthy skin, connective tissue, and gums and is the most widely taken vitamin supplement.

Vitamin C is vital in combating disease and healing muscle damage. It can also prevent the deterioration of other vitamins in the body, such as A, E, and some of the B vitamins. Vitamin C has been shown to help protect the bronchial airways and lungs from the effects of environmental toxins such as cold temperatures, pollens, smog, fumes, and chemicals. It is also said to protect against viral and bacterial infections, such as colds and flu, and to protect against radiation. Vitamin C is the primary antioxidant vitamin, preventing oxidation from damaging tissue. It is the most abundant antioxidant nutrient found in the lung's inner lining. Vitamin C can also help deal with some of the adverse effects of smoking by combating the oxidants, such as nitrogen oxide, which may be a cause of asthma in some people. The lungs of asthma sufferers are weakened from exposure to pollutants, contaminants, and oxidants, which can cause coughing, wheezing, and chest tightness. The more vitamin C they have, the better they can combat these symptoms. Seven studies conducted since 1973 have shown that asthma sufferers' breathing improves with vitamin C supplements.[6]

Clearly, the proper absorption and use of vitamin C is essential for asthmatics, and they need to be tested for sensitivity to it. As suggested earlier, sensitivity to vitamin C may cause many of the symptoms a person is trying to treat by taking the vitamin in the first place. For example, chronic sore throats may be caused by sensitivity to vitamin C, and taking the vitamin only makes the symptoms worse. After clearing for this sensitivity, the sore throat will disappear and vitamin C can be taken freely without the recurrence of symptoms.

People spend large amounts of money on vitamins recommended by health food stores, doctors, and other practitioners that may not be doing them any good. If people are sensitive to a vitamin, they will not be able to absorb and utilize it, no matter how much they take. Once sensitivity to vitamin C has been treated, people will begin to be able to extract it from their food. They will also be able to better utilize the nutrients from their foods without having to take excessive supplements.

Good food sources for vitamin C are tomatoes, citrus fruits, broccoli, strawberries, peppers, leafy greens, and potatoes. BioSET practitioners do both laboratory testing and muscle response testing to determine the best dosage for each individual. For people who are not sensitive to it, vitamin C is harmless, but it may increase toxicity in those who are sensitive and are not cleared for that sensitivity.

B VITAMINS

The B vitamin complex also presents problems for sensitive people. The complex is made up of at least eleven types of vitamins that are essential for the proper nourishment and functioning of our bodies. Almost everyone, however, is deficient in one or more B vitamins because it is difficult to get enough through a normal diet, especially when there is a high consumption of processed foods. Excessive sugar intake can also deplete B vitamins, since sugar contains no vitamins, minerals, or enzymes to aid in its digestion. By reducing the body's reserve of B vitamins, sugar actually decreases the available energy. High levels of caffeine deplete vitamin B, as do alcohol, stress, illness, and physical activity. We need a fresh supply of B complex vitamins every day because the body does not store them. Any excess is washed out through the kidneys or through perspiration.

The B vitamins include

- B1, thiamin
- B2, riboflavin
- B3, niacin or niacinamide
- B5, pantothenic acid
- B6, pyridoxine or pyridoxal-5-phosphate
- B12, cobalamin or cynocobalamin
- B9, folic acid or folacin
- PABA (para-aminobenzoic acid)
- B7, biotin
- Inositol
- Choline

These eleven vitamins are synergistic, which means they work as a team to perform all their vital individual functions properly and are more potent taken together than separately. Hence, many nutritionists recommend taking a B vitamin complex rather than single B vitamins. For proper metabolism of the B vitamins, the body must also maintain adequate levels of other nutrients such as iron and coenzymes. Thiamin, riboflavin, and niacin all bind to enzymes to help them do their job. None of these vitamins could function as effectively without their coenzymes. When clearing for B vitamin allergies, it is important to check all the vitamins, related nutrients, and coenzymes for sensitivity.

The primary function of B vitamins is to convert carbohydrates, fats, and proteins into energy the body can use. They are also vital for a properly functioning nervous system, producing red blood cells, maintaining muscle tone in the gastrointestinal tract, and healthy skin, hair, eyes, mouth, and liver. A high-potency vitamin B complex can help in recovering from debilitating illness, alcoholism, or excessive use of medication because it assists in reducing the effects of stress and supports the adrenal glands. Vitamin B supplementation is recommended for heavy coffee drinkers, women who take birth control pills, and people with high-carbohydrate diets.

Vitamin B1: Thiamin

Vitamin B1, or thiamin, aids in the digestion of carbohydrates, stabilizes the appetite, promotes growth and good muscle tone, inhibits pain, and assists in the normal functioning of the nervous system, muscles, and heart. Thiamin helps the body release energy from carbohydrates during metabolism. People who expend more energy and have high caloric intake need more thiamin than those who eat fewer calories. It can be depleted by excessive consumption of alcoholic beverages. A person deficient in vitamin B1 might experience a loss of appetite and weight, feelings of weakness and tiredness, paralysis, nervousness, irritability, insomnia, unfamiliar aches and pains, depression, heart difficulties, or constipation and gastrointestinal problems. A thiamin deficiency can also cause the disease beriberi, which results in weakness, nervous tingling of the body, and poor coordination. Good sources of thiamin are fruits, vegetables, and sunflower seeds.

Vitamin B2: Riboflavin

Vitamin B2, or riboflavin, is necessary for metabolizing carbohydrates, fats, and protein. Vitamin B2 also promotes general health by maintaining cell respiration, aiding in the formation of antibodies and red blood cells, ensuring good vision, relieving eye fatigue, and maintaining healthy nails and hair. The body's need for riboflavin may increase during periods of healing and pregnancy and in conditions such as asthma. A person deficient in vitamin B2 might experience sluggishness, itching and burning or bloodshot eyes, sores or cracks in and around the mouth and lips, a purplish or inflamed tongue and mouth, dermatitis, oily skin, slowed growth, trembling, digestive problems, and respiratory problems.

Good sources of riboflavin include dairy products, meat, poultry, and fish. To retain riboflavin during storage and cooking, food should be stored in containers that light cannot pass through, vegetables should be cooked in minimal amounts of water, and meat should be roasted or broiled.

Vitamin B3: Niacin

Vitamin B3, niacin or niacinamide, helps to improve the circulation and reduce the blood's cholesterol level. Vitamin B3 assists in maintaining the nervous system, tissue respiration, and fat synthesis and aids in metabolizing protein, sugar, and fat. It also helps the body do the following:

+ Reduce high blood pressure
+ Increase energy through the proper use of food
+ Produce acid
+ Metabolize sex hormones
+ Activate histamines
+ Prevent pellagra (a disease characterized by diarrhea and dermatitis)
+ Maintain healthy skin, tongue, and digestion

The body requires more niacin during periods of stress, acute illness, and low tryptophan intake.

Vitamin B3 is a good example of a vitamin that can be as effective as drugs in combating disease. Niacin, which is much less expensive than prescription medication, is successfully being used to lower levels of harmful cholesterol (LDL) and raise levels of good cholesterol (HDL).

A person deficient in vitamin B3 might experience gastrointestinal disturbance, loss of appetite, indigestion, bad breath, canker sores, skin disorders or rashes, muscular weakness, fatigue, insomnia, vague aches and pains, headaches, nervousness, memory loss, irritability, or depression. A deficiency can also result in respiratory problems including asthma, chronic bronchitis, or pellagra.

Niacin can be formed in the body from tryptophan, an essential amino acid. Good sources of niacin are mushrooms, asparagus, and peanuts. Loss of niacin from foods due to preparation and storage is slight, but vegetables should be cooked in a minimal amount of water and/or eaten raw.

Vitamin B5: Pantothenic Acid

Vitamin B5, or pantothenic acid, helps to release energy from carbohydrates, fats, and proteins; aids in the utilization of vitamins; and improves the body's resistance to stress. It also helps to do the following:

+ Build cells
+ Maintain the nervous system and the immune system
+ Maintain healthy skin
+ Support the adrenal glands in producing cortisone during times of stress

+ Fight infection by building antibodies
+ Detoxify the body
+ Stimulate growth
+ Utilize vitamin D

Vitamin B5 deficiencies can trigger asthmatic attacks, muscle cramping, painful and burning feet, skin abnormalities, retarded growth, dizzy spells, weakness, depression, decreased resistance to infection, restlessness, digestive disturbances, stomach stress, and vomiting. Vitamin B5 can be found in mushrooms, avocados, watermelon, pineapples, soy, lentils, bean sprouts, and peanuts.

Vitamin B6: Pyridoxine

Vitamin B6, pyridoxine or pyridoxal-5-phosphate, is necessary for synthesizing and breaking down DNA, RNA, and amino acids, the building blocks of protein, and the central nervous system requires it for normal brain functioning. Vitamin B6 also aids in metabolizing fat and carbohydrates, forming antibodies, and removing excess fluid and discomfort during a menstrual period. It aids hemoglobin in its function; promotes healthy skin; reduces muscle spasms, leg cramps, and stiffness in the hands; helps to prevent nausea; and promotes the balance of sodium and phosphorus in the body.

Conditions that respond to vitamin B6 therapy include carpal tunnel syndrome, joint pain, homocystinuria (a hereditary disease leading to the accumulation of homocysteine in the urine), sensitivity to bright light, sensitivity to MSG, burning or tingling in the extremities, the inability to recall dreams, and imbalances of the liver. Because the body uses vitamin B6 to break down protein, the more protein one eats, the more vitamin B6 one needs. Deficiencies can produce skin eruptions of dermatitis, loss of muscular control or muscle weakness, arm and leg cramps, fatigue, nervousness, irritability, insomnia, slow learning, water retention, anemia, mouth disorders, or hair loss.

Fruits and vegetables are good sources of vitamin B6. To retain vitamin B6 during cooking, serve fruits raw and cook vegetables in minimal amounts of water for the shortest time possible.

Vitamin B12: Cobalamin

Vitamin B12, cobalamin or cynocobalamin, is required for forming and regenerating red blood cells to help prevent anemia. Vitamin B12 is also necessary for building genetic material; metabolizing carbohydrates, fat, and protein; increasing energy; and maintaining a healthy nervous system and muscles. It is important for promoting DNA synthesis in childhood growth, cell longevity, memory improvement, maintaining the appetite and digestive system, and strengthening the immune system. It aids in the absorption of iron and calcium and helps prevent inflammation. It also assists in metabolizing folic acid and in synthesizing DNA, and it is essential for producing insulation for nerve fibers. Vitamin B12 and a coenzyme combine to form a substance called dibencozide, which aids in the conversion of fat to lean muscle tissue. For this reason, many strength athletes, such as weight lifters, take vitamin B12 as a safe, competitive, and legal alternative to steroid hormones. A vitamin B12–folate complex can be used as a tonic to assist in converting iron to hemoglobin, helping normalize hormonal production, and improving short-term memory in the elderly. Vitamin B12 is even considered an antiaging nutrient and an agent for increasing sperm count. Sufficient levels of vitamin B12 are considered especially crucial for women during pregnancy and lactation.

There is some controversy today about the best way to get enough vitamin B12 in one's diet. Some experts claim that vitamin B12 is only acquired naturally by eating meat, eggs, and milk products, but vegetarians and vegans claim they have found numerous nonanimal sources of this vital nutrient, including edible seaweed such as hijiki and wakame, certain mushrooms, tofu, tempeh, miso, and parsley. Some nutritionists disagree, saying that the only sources of vitamin B12 available to vegetarians are fortified nutritional yeast, fortified breakfast cereals, soy milk, and other soy products.

Supplements that contain spirulina or nori (another seaweed) can interfere with vitamin B12 absorption. Some experts also advise against taking multivitamin products because these preparations may contain products that interfere with the breakdown of vitamin B12. By preventing the absorption of vitamin B12, they help to create the deficiency they are supposed to correct.

A person deficient in vitamin B12 could experience pernicious (life-threatening) anemia, degeneration of the spinal cord and nerves, poor appetite, stunted growth (in children), nervousness, depression, a lack of balance, neuritis (a nerve impairment), or brain damage. Symptoms of anemia may include a pale and yellow, sallow complexion; a shiny or red, sore tongue; weakness and fatigue progressing to paralysis; numbness or tingling in the hands and feet; a gradual deterioration of motor coordination; moodiness; poor memory and confusion; even delirium, delusion, hallucinations, and psychotic states. Paralysis and possible death may occur with the deterioration of myelin sheaths (which insulate nerve cells) and the failure of DNA production.

A vitamin B12 deficiency, especially among the elderly, may occur even though the person's diet contains enough vitamin B12 because other substances needed for vitamin B12 absorption may be lacking. For example, the stomach manufactures something known as the "intrinsic factor," which must bond with vitamin B12 before the body can absorb it. Other substances that are needed for absorption include iron, folic acid, and a factor manufactured in the stomach, which intestinal parasites can block. Microorganisms in the stomach can compete for the vitamin B12, and toxins can block absorption. Enzyme deficiencies, liver or kidney disease, and atrophic gastritis can interfere with the utilization of vitamin B12.

Vitamin B12 can be further depleted by disease, hypothyroidism, and a sensitivity to lactose. Consumption of foods such as meat and animal products, refined sugars, carbohydrates, drugs, chemicals, caffeine, alcoholic beverages, tobacco, megadoses of vitamin C, egg albumen, egg yoke, and allergies to any of those can all use up the body's store of vitamin B12.

Vitamin B12 can be produced by bacterial activity in the body's own small intestines, mouth, teeth, gums, nasal passages, and around the tonsils, tongue, and upper bronchial tree. Since vitamin B12 is often found in soil, freshly picked raw, unwashed vegetables, especially root vegetables, may have vitamin B12 on their surfaces. To retain the vitamin B12 in meat or fish, they should be roasted or broiled.

Folic Acid

Folic acid (folate or folacin) helps the body produce red blood cells and form genetic material within every cell in the body. Folic acid also works with vitamin B12 in synthesizing DNA and RNA, which is essential for the growth and reproduction of all body cells. It is useful in converting amino acids, breaking down and assimilating protein, stimulating the appetite, maintaining a healthy intestinal tract, and forming nucleonic acid. Folic acid may reverse certain types of anemia, reduce the risk of cervical displasia, and lower the likelihood of heart attack. It becomes even more essential during times of growth and cell reproduction, especially during pregnancy, when folic acid seems to be in short supply. It can protect unborn babies from neural tube defects and other midline birth anomalies.

Folic acid deficiency during pregnancy can cause the disease spina bifida in the child, which can be permanently crippling. Recently it was discovered that folic acid reduces the risk of premature birth. Deficiency can result in megaloblastic anemia, in which red blood cells fail to divide properly, becoming large and abnormal and causing a shortage of red blood cells. Other symptoms of folic acid deficiency are gastrointestinal disorders, prematurely gray hair, a pale tongue, and vitamin B12 deficiency.

Good sources of folic acid include fruits and vegetables, especially citrus fruits, tomatoes, leafy greens, cooked spinach, lettuce, broccoli, and organ meats. To retain folic acid, fruits and vegetables should be served raw, if possible, or steamed or simmered in a minimal amount of water. Always store vegetables in the refrigerator to keep them fresh.

PABA

Para-aminobenzoic acid (PABA) is a component of folic acid as well as an antioxidant and cell membrane stabilizer. It helps to prevent red blood cells from bursting and lysosomal membranes (which contain digestive enzymes) from breaking and releasing tissue-damaging enzymes. PABA helps bacteria to produce folic acid, and it aids in forming red blood cells and assimilating pantothenic acid (vitamin B5). It produces healthy skin and skin pigmentation, helps return gray hair to its natural color, and screens the skin from sun exposure. A PABA deficiency may cause extreme fatigue, irritability, depression, nervousness, eczema, constipation, digestive disorders, headaches, and premature graying of hair. Good sources of PABA include liver, kidney, mushrooms, leafy greens, spinach, molasses, and brewer's yeast.

Biotin

Biotin helps to strengthen the immune system; aids in the utilization of protein, folic acid, pantothenic acid, and vitamin B12; aids in cell growth, fatty acid production, and synthesis; helps to form DNA and RNA; and helps to produce healthy hair.

Anyone who is sensitive to this B vitamin will not be able to properly absorb it or the other B vitamins; therefore, this sensitivity could produce a deficiency in *all* the B vitamins. A biotin deficiency may lead to drowsiness, extreme exhaustion, depression, loss of appetite, muscle pain, and gray skin color. Good sources of biotin include soy, liver, kidney, brewer's yeast, milk, molasses, fruit, nuts, beef, and egg yolk.

Inositol

Inositol, found in every cell of the body, is necessary for growing muscle cells and forming lecithin. It helps break down fats, reduce blood cholesterol, and prevent thinning hair. Inositol is also an antioxidant free radical scavenger and is known as "nature's tranquilizer" for the calming effect it often has. A deficiency may result in hair loss, eczema, constipation, migraines, and high blood cholesterol.

Choline

Choline is very important in controlling fat and cholesterol buildup in the body, preventing fat from accumulating in the liver, and facilitating the movement of fats in the cells and throughout the bloodstream. It also helps regulate the kidneys, liver, and gallbladder and is important to the health of myelin sheaths, which cover the nerve fibers, and to nerve transmission. Choline is known to help improve memory and support brain chemistry and is an essential component of acetylcholine, an important neurotransmitter.

A deficiency in choline may result in cirrhosis and fatty degeneration of the liver, hardening of the arteries, heart problems, high blood pressure, and hemorrhaging kidneys. Good sources of choline include brewer's yeast, egg yolks, liver, leafy greens, legumes, peas, beans, heart, and lecithin. Choline should be taken with the other B vitamins for optimal effectiveness.

Clearing Sensitivities to B Vitamins

Sensitivities to B vitamins are among the most important to clear with Bio-SET because many foods have high B vitamin content. Eating vitamin-rich foods and taking supplements can do more harm than good to B vitamin-sensitive people. For asthmatics, the most common problems are with vitamin B2 (riboflavin), vitamin B5, vitamin B6 (pyridoxine), and vitamin B12 (cobalamin). Other B vitamins, or all of them, may be causing difficulty. If a client has asthma and other chronic problems, BioSET practitioners test for each of the B vitamins separately.

Eczema is often a precursor to asthma, and BioSET practitioners have found that sensitivities to vitamins B and C are closely connected to eczema, especially in young children. BioSET has been very effective in eradicating eczema and decreasing the likelihood of asthma.

Possible symptoms of B vitamin deficiency are mood swings, behavioral problems, cold sores, herpes, extreme fatigue, severe bloating, malnutrition, chronic sinus congestion, and chronic yeast infection. Chronic yeast infections may often involve B vitamin sensitivities and deficiencies, and clearing for B vitamins can sometimes take care of these health problems.

VITAMIN E

Vitamin E is a fat-soluble antioxidant that protects cells from free radical damage and neutralizes the damaging effects of ozone. Since asthmatics tend to worsen after ozone exposure, this can be a key nutrient for them.

VITAMIN A

Vitamin A comes in two forms, beta carotene, which is found in a wide variety of fruits and vegetables, and vitamin A itself, which is found in liver, eggs, cod liver oil, butter, and dairy products. Recent research suggests that beta carotene, which is known to be a precursor to vitamin A, can boost the immune system and prevent arteries from clogging. Beta carotene and vitamin A are both fat-soluble vitamins. Vitamin A is important for eyesight, healthy skin, a healthy intestinal tract, and protection against the free radicals caused in the body by exposure to pollutants. This supplement is important in strengthening the immune system and protecting against infection. High doses of vitamin A can help fight viral infections and are effective in combating illnesses and treating wounds.

Excessive consumption of alcohol, and the resulting liver damage, can deplete vitamin A. When your liver is impaired, you are not able to metabolize vitamin A and several other nutrients. Smoking also depletes vitamin A in the respiratory tract.

Because vitamin A is retained in the body, it is important not to take excessively high doses that can build up to a toxic level. A sensitivity check should always be done before taking supplements.

BioSET practitioners have cleared many people, especially children, for sensitivity to vitamin A. This sensitivity is significant in children who have chronic coughs, chronic infections involving the respiratory system, and asthma.

Food sources for vitamin A include papayas, peaches, and other yellow fruit, as well as asparagus, beets, broccoli, carrots, Swiss chard, kale, turnip greens, watercress, parsley, red peppers, sweet potatoes, squash, pumpkin, corn, and spirulina. People with low thyroid have trouble converting beta carotene to vitamin A and require a regular intake of vitamin A through food or supplements. Beta carotene is found in deep green vegetables like spinach and broccoli, sweet potatoes, carrots, squash (especially winter squash), grapefruit, mangoes, and apricots. These foods are also full of vitamin C and other antioxidants.

VITAMIN F

Essential fatty acids help to build cell membranes, support the nervous system, and boost the immune system to help ward off disease. Fat also helps slow the release of sugar into the bloodstream, so they are important for those who are hypoglycemic or diabetic. Fat is needed to absorb vitamins A, D, and K and beta carotene.

Of all the fats we consume, there are only two essential fatty acids, omega-6 fatty acid (linoleic) and omega-3 fatty acid (alpha linolenic). Eating junk food, including fat-free health store junk food, depletes your stores of essential fatty acids. Eating fried foods, margarine, and vegetable shortening can cause rancidity of oils and should be avoided.

Omega-6 can be found in all vegetable oils and most beans. Omega-3 is found in fewer foods: flaxseed, flax oil, fresh walnuts, walnut oil, pumpkin seeds, and soy and canola oils. It is important to buy oils that are not refined or rancid and to avoid buying oils sold in clear glass bottles in supermarkets. Always buy oils stored in dark brown bottles because light exposure causes them to spoil.

Because good fat metabolism is key to proper use of essential fatty acids, I use enzyme therapy to ensure absorption of the good fatty acids from a regular diet (see chapter 13). This works well in combination with BioSET clearings for any sensitivity to fatty acids or the foods containing them.

MINERALS

Common minerals to which people may be sensitivite include silver, gold, copper, vanadium, potassium, sulfur, copper, chromium, and magnesium. A deficiency of magnesium, which is the most important mineral for asthmatics, can increase the amount of histamine released from cells, causing constriction of the bronchioles and triggering the onset of asthma. Magnesium is a specific smooth-muscle relaxant and can work magically to eliminate severe acute asthma attacks. It is also a natural laxative and, therefore, helpful for people with chronic constipation. Large doses are safe with many asthmatic medications.

A study from Britain tested over 2,500 adults with a chemical that can cause constricted airways in asthmatics. They found that people with low magnesium diets were twice as likely to have an asthmatic reaction as those with high magnesium diets.[7] This study spurred further research into the anti-inflammatory properties of magnesium.

This study also prompted me to test asthmatics for sensitivity to magnesium and to foods high in magnesium, such as seafood, whole grains, dark green vegetables, molasses, nuts, and bonemeal. As it turns out, many asthmatics are sensitive to magnesium and respond well to treatment for this mineral. One asthmatic man came to see me with chronic sinus infections and respiratory problems. After he was cleared for his sensitivity to minerals, especially magnesium, and began supplementing with 1,000 to 1,500 mg of magnesium per day, he had far fewer asthma symptoms and his reactions were less frequent. He has not used an inhaler or any other medication now for over two years.

For infants and children, BioSET practitioners suggest a supplement with a liquid magnesium, which we have found is well tolerated—about one teaspoon for each twenty pounds of body weight. As with other supplements, we always test the individual to find out how much of the supplement is needed.

ANTIOXIDANTS

Unfortunately, people can have a sensitivity to antioxidants, which is especially problematic for asthmatics. Antioxidants are known as free radical scavengers because they remove dangerous free radical particles from the tissue, thereby strengthening the immune system, building up tissue, and regenerating the body. They are particularly important for anyone with a chronic illness. The basic antioxidants are vitamins C and E, the B vitamins, fatty acids, and beta carotene. New antioxidants are being discovered all the time, including zinc, copper, selenium, N-acetylcysteine (NAC), glutamine, and choline. BioSET practitioners test and treat for each of these because they are so important to good health. Once people are cleared of their sensitivities to antioxidants, they should be able to derive them easily from eating a good diet, since antioxidants are plentiful in many foods.

N-ACETYLCYSTEINE (NAC)

One antioxidant worth discussing in greater detail is N-acetylcysteine (NAC), an amino acid and building block for glutathione, one of the most powerful free radical scavengers in the body. Glutathione helps the liver detoxify medications, which can be particularly helpful for asthmatics on large amounts of medication. The immune systems of many asthma patients have been compromised by large doses of chemicals, such as cortisone and prednisone, and they need help in detoxifying their immune system and building up their energy and stamina. Good sources of N-acetylcysteine include poultry, yogurt, egg yolks, garlic, onions, red peppers, broccoli, and brussels sprouts.

SELENIUM

Selenium, a trace mineral, is another building block of glutathione and is therefore important for detoxification. Selenium also helps vitamin E prevent free radical damage. Good sources of selenium include fish, shellfish, red meat, grains, eggs, chicken, liver, brewer's yeast, and garlic.

Enzyme Deficiencies Caused by Sensitivities

Enzyme deficiencies are another little-known cause of asthma.

AMYLASE

After conducting enzyme evaluations, BioSET practitioners find that many of their asthmatic patients are extremely deficient in amylase (see chapter 13 for more discussion). Since amylase is an important anti-inflammatory, people who are deficient in amylase are not properly fighting against environmental pollutants and allergens that cause irritation to the lungs and respiratory system. In combination with other enzymes, amylase is important in digesting carbohydrates. BioSET practitioners have found that a deficiency in amylase is often linked to a sensitivity to amylase and the enzyme amylopsin. Clearing for this sensitivity, then supplementing with the enzymes can be very helpful.

PROTEASE

Protease is another enzyme that is critical in treating asthma. It is important for digesting protein and as a natural antibiotic, anti-infectant, and anti-inflammatory agent. It can help fight pathogens, repair tissue damage, regenerate tissue, remove tissue debris, and break down foreign bodies that the immune system might identify as allergens or pathogens.

Much of the vulnerability to infections that asthmatics suffer is due to a deficiency of protease. Once the sensitivity is cleared, BioSET practitioners suggest high doses of a protease supplement.

CORTISONE

Cortisone, a synthetic version of cortisol, is commonly used as an anti-inflammatory for asthmatics as well as for other chronic conditions, such as MS and rheumatoid arthritis. People who are sensitive to their own cortisol may also be sensitive to cortisone, causing serious reactions. A study done on seventy-six patients who were treated with cortisone showed that cortisone therapy tended to cause an inability to digest carbohydrates, which may have been due to a deficiency of amylase. Cortisone can also cause a worsening of gastroduodenal ulcers and can cause bleeding and even perforation of the intestinal lining. Women over fifty tend to have reflux and gastritis, and cortisone therapy can worsen these conditions.

Gastric problems can be helped with several supplements and enzymes, including marshmallow root extract, aloe vera juice extract, deglycyrrhizenated licorice root extract, and amylase, lipase, cellulase, lactase, invertase, peptidase, alpha galactosidase, or glucoamylase.

Cortisone clearing and therapy also lessens a patient's resistance to infection, which can result in fever, malaise, chronic bronchitis, and sinusitis in asthmatics. Many asthmatics who have been on prednisone and corticosteroids or hydrocortisone therapy for some time are deficient in the enzyme protease, which is a natural anti-inflammatory. Supplementing with protease helps them fight infections and deal with inflammation naturally. The enzyme inhibits inflammation without suppressing amino acids, as steroids do, and improves blood circulation and nutrition of the tissue.

Many people with chronic health problems such as fatigue, asthma, and rheumatoid arthritis do extremely well with enzyme therapy. The most noticeable results are with asthmatics who have problems with chronic infections. They generally come in with recurring bronchitis, always on antibiotics, never looking well, never having enough energy. After enzyme therapy they are able to fight infections without using antibiotics and have far fewer asthmatic episodes without steroid therapy. They are happier, feel and look better, and do not age as quickly.

One asthmatic patient of mine was traveling with a friend who showed signs of infection. The patient treated herself for her saliva with BioSET using the acupressure points she had learned and then increased her protease and antioxidant intake. She was able to resist the infection without using antibiotics, which she had been unable to do in the past.

Metabolic Imbalances

A healthy metabolism is vital for limiting various sensitivities. Metabolic imbalances can aggravate or even cause asthma in some people.

THE IMPORTANCE OF DETOXIFICATION

One of the primary causes of metabolic imbalance is the toxicity resulting from a body's inability to rid itself of metabolic waste products. This condition is worsened by incomplete oxidation in the tissues, poor nutrition, and resulting chronic disease. The liver, which is the organ primarily responsible for eliminating toxins, is severely stressed by prolonged treatment with cortisone, prednisone, antibiotics, inhalers, and other medications. Other organs responsible for detoxification include the skin, intestines, kidneys, and lungs.

Good blood and lymph circulation is also important for detoxification. The blood supplies oxygen and nutrients to the cells and also cleanses, transports, and disposes of metabolic waste through excretion via the intestines, kidneys, lungs, and skin. In the lymph system, macrophages, which are the body's first line of defense against infection, travel around eating up foreign substances and breaking them down into smaller, nontoxic components. Well-functioning macrophages are essential for the effective elimination of pathogens, metabolic waste, and toxins.

In a healthy immune system, antibodies and lymphocytes are present in the blood and lymph and immediately recognize foreign cells, such as bacteria, viruses, fungi, and toxic waste. They bind with these substances to form immune complexes that the macrophages can degrade and eat up. When a small number of immune complexes are present, the macrophages can easily consume them before they do harm. But when an overabundance of immune complexes are present or the macrophages are inhibited by medications and metabolic waste, these complexes affix themselves to body tissue. This calls the secondary backup immune defenses into play, which may cause autoimmune inflammation and, ultimately, chronic degenerative disorders such as asthma, rheumatoid arthritis, or thyroid disease.

These immune complex diseases will not occur as long as macrophages retain their ability to function properly. Many metabolic toxins and addictive substances, such as cocaine, morphine, steroids, and cortisone, inhibit macrophage activity and thus contribute to immune complex disease. Certain enzyme mixtures are effective in removing and preventing immune complexes and keeping macrophage activity intact. Clearing chronic degenerative disorders caused by circulating immune complexes with enzymes and BioSET can result in improved appetite, reduced depression, and decreased inflammation.

LIVER TOXICITY

The liver, which is the principal organ of detoxification, eliminates inhaled and ingested substances and other toxic compounds and drug by-products from the gastrointestinal organs. Many factors contribute to liver toxicity: drug reactions, pesticides, hormones, inhaled toxic substances, food sensitivities, and genetic disposition. Genetically determined enzyme processes may vary and influence an individual's ability to detoxify. For example, risk for smoking-induced cancer and other health problems will depend in part on one's genetic detoxification system. Individuals who cannot adequately detoxify the hydrocarbons in cigarette smoke have increased risks for smoking-induced cancers. Exposure to fat-soluble toxins, pesticides, and alcohol may also increase the risk of liver damage by depleting important antioxidants and increasing oxidant-induced damage. Oxygen free radicals play a significant role in promoting and progressing liver diseases. Metabolites from gut bacteria as well as substances like sulfites, naturally occurring compounds in foods that are used as food additives, can deter liver detoxification and contribute to liver damage.

By clearing sensitivities and improving digestion and immune function, BioSET can help spare the liver unnecessary toxicity. In addition, there are many good liver detoxification programs utilizing supplements and nutrients, such as the amino acids, vitamin B5 (pantothenic acid), certain hepatic coenzymes, glutathione, and sulfates. These help rid the liver of drugs, food additives, environmental pollutants, and steroid hormones. Recent studies have shown that people with chronic fatigue, fibromyalgia, multiple chemical sensitivities, and asthma suffer metabolic toxicity and imbalance and, therefore, benefit from such programs.

CORRECTING METABOLIC IMBALANCES IN ASTHMATICS

To correct metabolic imbalances in asthmatics, it is important to facilitate the excretion and elimination of metabolic waste and toxins from the body. Asthmatics are often constipated, experience chronic loose stools, or fluctuate between the two. They may also suffer bloating and poor food absorption. These problems are usually caused by sugar and starch intolerance and poor digestion. BioSET practitioners use enzymes to treat this condition, rather than more invasive therapies such as enemas or colonics.

While facilitating proper intestinal elimination, BioSET practitioners also make sure the kidneys are working properly. They can be stimulated by increasing liquid intake, using herbs such as horsetail and goldenrod, and prescribing enzymes for optimal kidney detoxification. The herbs are mild diuretics that stimulate kidney function. Exercise and diet are also important, as is the process of clearing food sensitivities and avoiding highly toxic foods such as alcohol, caffeine, and excess salt.

The skin is also an important organ of elimination, and skin brushing is one method for helping the skin detoxify. Using a firm, hard vegetable brush, brush your skin vigorously for five minutes before you take a shower in the morning. Foods that can clog or toxify the skin are food allergens, dairy products, and highly fatty foods. Foods that help the skin with elimination are those high in enzymes and vitamins A and E, such as wheat germ oil and beta-carotene.

Chiropractic Misalignments and Myofascitis

When I first began to practice chiropractic, I treated a young man who had suffered from asthma his whole life. He complained of chronic stiffness and spasm in his upper back and neck (myofascitis). When I examined him, I found some chronic spinal misalignments at the levels of T1–7 (thoracic), with extreme mild fascitis, or inflamed soft tissue. Since the nerves from these particular vertebrae enervate the lung and heart area, I thought that relaxing the muscles in the area, increasing his flexibility, and aligning the vertebrae might help his respiration as well. I was right. After a series of treatments, his asthma improved so much that he no longer required any medication or treatment. Over the years I have often had positive results with chiropractic care for asthma and other lung-related problems. Also, there are certain points on the spine where tapping with the fingers or with certain tools will open up the bronchioles and relieve an asthmatic attack.

In a recent study, children with asthma showed an overall improvement in lung capacity after only fifteen chiropractic adjustments.[8] There is ample research documenting the intimate connection between the spinal column, the nervous system, and the respiratory system. It has also been shown that vertebral subluxation in the neck and upper back can produce muscle spasms that can cause lymphatic congestion. With the lymph system unable to dispose of bacteria, debris, and other foreign materials, toxins will accumulate in the area. In many cases, chiropractic adjustments will produce immediate relaxation of the neck and back muscles, thereby increasing lymphatic drainage, improving respiratory function, and helping to cleanse the system and improve immunity.

The chiropractic approach to health care is safe and natural and can benefit children and adults of all ages.

Asthma: Emotional or Psychosomatic?

One question that clients often ask me is, can emotional distress bring on an asthma attack? Absolutely. One female asthmatic I treated became free of symptoms after she divorced her husband. A man's asthmatic symptoms disappeared when his father died of cancer after a long and painful illness. Another patient stopped having asthma attacks after being treated for sorrow related to an incident with her mother that had happened almost thirty years before.

Over the years I have developed a deep respect for our emotions and the power dramatic life events have to affect our health. Many people suffering from migraines, digestive problems, chronic fatigue, or joint problems need to do emotional clearing. Every asthmatic I have treated has needed to clear certain emotional blockages as part of the path to healing and regeneration. Problems or symptom complexes inevitably involve unresolved emotions.

Fortunately, emotional clearing is possible with BioSET. BioSET unlocks the energy around traumas and helps to clear it from the body so that it will not continue to create energy blockages and health problems. Many emotional blockages are easily cleared or worked through during treatment of one's basic sensitivities, but some traumas and repressed emotions need to be confronted, felt, and then released from the body and nervous system. These emotions can be connected with food cravings, eating disorders, and environmental factors, as well as with family members, friends, and loved ones. The emotions can be related to love, intimacy, finances, health, physical or emotional abuse, rape, or molestation. And they can be rooted in specific incidents such as the death of a loved one or a divorce. They may also arise out of a recurring pattern of events, such as fighting at the dinner table, financial stress, marital difficulties, or repeated abuse. Minor, seemingly petty incidents in childhood can create serious sensitivities or blockages in the energy pathways that act as triggers for asthmatics. In Chinese medicine, sorrow is related to the lungs; therefore, it is no surprise that sorrow is a common emotion found among asthmatics or that asthmatics respond dramatically to treatments for sorrow. Emotions are often the primary cause of asthma attacks.

Children are especially sensitive to emotional clearings. I have seen children with chronic coughs immediately stop coughing during a clearing of a sensitivity. One little girl was having a rough time being weaned. Several months after I treated her for sensitivities to mother's milk, she weaned herself naturally with no emotional upset and no pressure from her parents. A boy who was having trouble with his writing turned out to be afraid of his teacher. When we cleared him for his sensitivity to wheat, he was able to express his fear, and from then on his problems disappeared.

Never underestimate the power of emotions and their relation to food sensitivities or the seriousness of the illnesses they can produce. Many food sensitivities are the result of emotional experiences with food. A man with chronic bloating, indigestion, and fatigue was discovered to have unresolved shame in relation to his parents. Within days of being cleared for his sensitivity to certain vegetables, his symptoms disappeared. That is why it is important to have calm surroundings when one eats. If people eat when they are angry, for example, they may develop a sensitivity to foods eaten at that time. I always tell my patients, "Please don't eat when you're upset, and please don't argue during a meal." Even positive emotions of elation can create sensitivities. A meal is a sacred event and should be peaceful, like meditation. Leave any discussion of intense issues until after the meal is finished.

People often ask me to have lunch with them, but I always take a rain check. To avoid creating sensitivities through emotional situations or discussions during a meal, I would rather eat at home in a quiet, soothing surrounding. Many of my meals at home as a youngster were emotionally charged. No wonder I had poor digestion and extensive food sensitivities for most of my life! Now I insist on eating with serenity and awareness, and I recommend that my patients do the same.

Stress

Stress is another important factor in the incidence of asthma. I believe that if people have good health, a strong immune system, an adequately functioning liver, and good digestion, they will not be physically vulnerable to the stresses they encounter every day of their lives. If, however, they have many hidden sensitivities, poor digestion, poor eating habits, poor immune function, high levels of immune complexes, and liver toxicity, they will be susceptible to stress, which will add just one more strain to an already overburdened system and increase the likelihood of illness, including asthma. The best way to manage stress and avoid the physical consequences that often ensue is to strengthen the immune system and overall health.

Stress affects people of all ages, including infants, children, and the elderly. Whether the stress is being weaned from the breast, learning to write in school, or going through difficult life changes, everyone needs to strengthen their immune system to help their body resist the effects of stress. This is my goal for each individual, and I find that enzyme therapy, elimination of food and environmental sensitivities, proper diet, exercise, and the maintenance of spiritual and mental good health are all important factors.

Troubleshooting and Preventive Measures for Asthma Sufferers

Many people with asthma do not know what causes the disease or triggers their attacks. They may be doing fine for a period of days or weeks or even months, and then suddenly, within a period of hours, they begin to feel a tightness and heaviness in their chest, they find it difficult to breathe, and they start to cough or wheeze. Sometimes they have to go to the hospital emergency room for treatment with steroids. "I know it's probably related to sensitivities," they tell me, "but I'm not sure which sensitivities are the worst. What can I do? How can I know why my body is reacting the way it is? And how can I eliminate the sensitivities that are the most severe and causing the most irritation to my lungs?"

Diagnostic Evaluation

When a person first sees a BioSET practitioner, the practitioner does some preliminary work to help find an answer to these questions. First the practitioner conducts a BioSET meridian toxicity evaluation, then a complete enzyme evaluation and a common food sensitivity test, with and without accounting for the related digestive enzymes. Lastly, there is an evaluation of some basic environmental sensitivities, which were discussed in chapter 1. Additionally, the person is requested to keep a diary of their asthma symptoms, their daily diet in detail, what supplements they take, and so on. With this information, the assessment can begin.

For example, a practitioner may find indications of various sensitivities that could be having a major impact on or creating inflammation in the body. When pointed out, a patient can then note in their diary whether, for example, eating dairy increases mucus or causes symptoms such as sinus congestion that could be precursors to an asthmatic episode. The person can also determine whether their sensitivities are mainly to food, environmental toxins, or both.

Clearing basic sensitivities with BioSET will often eliminate many other sensitivities as well, which may significantly reduce an asthmatic's need for medication. At this point it becomes easier to spot additional allergens that may be causing trouble. One woman who came to see me had asthma episodes her entire life. There were times when she was fine, but sometimes her attacks were so serious they became life threatening and she ended up in the hospital. "Why does this happen?" she wanted to know. "What is the real cause of my asthma? I know it's sensitivity related, but what sensitivities are the cause? Is it environmental? I'm a gardener and I'm outside all the time. Is it the flowers, the food, my house, mold, smoke? Sometimes these things bother me, and sometimes I seem to be OK with them. I'm confused." She also suffered from sinusitis and chronic sinus congestion.

I began by doing a routine evaluation. I found toxicity in her liver and gallbladder. I also noticed indications of systemic candida and other fungi, an inability to digest or absorb sugars, and hypoadrenal indicators. This was not surprising because the adrenal gland is intimately involved with inflammation, metabolizing sugars, and regulating energy levels in the body. I also noticed that the woman was a little constipated. After reviewing her diet, I had a better understanding of her situation. She was sugar intolerant, and her consumption of large amounts of sugar was weakening and compromising her immune system. I recommended a diet with far fewer carbohydrates than the diet she was accustomed to following. I also prescribed enzymes for digesting sugars, enzymes for relieving nasal congestion, and enzymes to support her liver and reduce toxicity. Through testing, I found that she had many of the basic common sensitivities, including several food sensitivities. Her most severe sensitivities, though, were to environmental substances: pollen, dust, mold, smuts and rust, grains, grain dust, rugs, paints, smoke, perfumes, and other inhalants. I treated her for her basic sensitivities and then for her environmental sensitivities.

Health Plan

Good health starts with a solid plan. This section will help you create a plan specifically suited to your health needs and goals.

KEEPING A DIARY

After embarking on a low-sugar diet, this woman began keeping a diary to record what she ate, how she felt each day, and what sensitivity symptoms she experienced. After her initial clearing, her symptoms were greatly reduced, and she became much more aware of which foods and substances she was sensitive to and was able to avoid them. She realized certain foods caused congestion and coughing, certain environmental factors caused wheezing and tightness, and certain fungi and contactants created sinus congestion. Through self-diagnosis (muscle testing), she was able to ascertain which particular infectants were the most problematic and needed to be treated and cleared. She progressed well with her treatments, and we managed to clear her essential sensitivities. Today she is doing extremely well and rarely has an asthmatic episode.

It is important that both the patient and the practitioner act as detectives. From long experience working with asthma patients, BioSET practitioners can usually determine which sensitivities are the most serious for a particular patient, but everyone is different. Patients need to know what they are digesting and not digesting, absorbing and not absorbing, and what they are deficient in so adjustments can be made. They need to become more aware of what they are bombarded with in their everyday lives and which substances provoke reactions.

Most patients, even children, become excellent detectives. They say, "I know that it was the food additive I ate that triggered the asthma," or "I know it was pollen, or chocolate, or perfume, or something in my room." They get to know their own bodies, and BioSET practitioners listen to what they report.

EATING SMART

Food sensitivities can be serious triggers for asthma. The most common trigger foods include

- Alcohol
- Baking powder
- Baking soda
- Caffeine
- Chocolate
- Citrus fruits
- Coffee
- Corn
- Cow's milk

- Eggplant
- Grains, most
- Gum mix
- Nuts, various
- Onions
- Peppers
- Potatoes
- Seeds
- Spices
- Soy and soy products
- Tomatoes
- Wheat
- Yeast products

Plants that contain gluten, such as wheat, rye, oats, malt, and barley, also contribute to asthma symptoms.

Since most asthmatics are sugar intolerant, BioSET practitioners usually recommend a reduction in their intake of sugars and carbohydrates. For those who are not, we make dietary recommendations specific to their needs. Since dairy products are highly mucus forming, as are apple juice, bananas, and chocolate, we routinely suggest avoiding these foods until the patient is cleared, then suggest adding them back into the diet slowly, if at all.

Both pesticides and hormones can cause problems for asthmatics also, so practitioners recommend organically grown fruits, vegetables, and grains, as well as organically raised, hormone-free meats as much as possible. Pesticides, nitrates, food additives, and hormones can often be found in red meat, chicken, and other poultry and should be avoided whenever possible. It is important for asthmatics to learn what foods they are sensitive to and then avoid them or be cleared for them. To get rid of pesticides from fruits and vegetables, scrub them with natural products, such as grapefruit extract and borax. Some health food stores even sell fruit and vegetable washing solutions.

Sulfites are added as a preservative in foods such as wine, beer, fruit drinks, cider, certain baked products, gelatin, starches, beet sugar, and dried fruits, and to prevent discoloration in fresh shrimp, raw vegetables, and salads. Buying foods with less packaging and processing can help alleviate the harmful effects of sulfites and other food additives.

One patient who came to see me had improved so much over a year of treatments that she could do without her medication for months at a time.

Then, while at a restaurant, she inadvertently ate a dish containing foods for which she had not been treated. She had such a severe reaction that she had to use her inhaler. Asthmatics should know what they are eating, where it comes from, how it is cooked, and with what other ingredients it is cooked. Otherwise, cooking at home from scratch is probably the safest approach until most allergens are cleared.

TAKING DIETARY SUPPLEMENTS

For dietary supplementation BioSET practitioners recommend taking digestive enzymes with each meal, and taking systemic enzymes in between meals, which include various vitamins and minerals or herbs, to control inflammation. Of course, a person is always checked to make sure they are not sensitive to a supplement before taking it. Different brands of supplements have different fillers in them, and people need to be checked for each one before taking it. When people first come to see a BioSET practitioner, they are encouraged to bring all of their supplements, and they are checked to see if they are sensitive to any one of them. After a person is cleared for any sensitivities to vitamins and minerals, they often supplement their diet with these nutrients, in a combination formula with enzymes that enhance their absorption into each cell. This will usually make up for deficiencies a patient may have as a result of their former sensitivities.

For example, sensitivity to calcium often indicates a deficiency of calcium, which will be revealed in the sensitivity testing. After clearing a person for the sensitivity, I will recommend a calcium supplement in an enzyme formula to help the body optimally absorb the calcium from the foods they eat. Before they begin taking it, I will test to see how much supplementation they need.

An asthmatic named Patti came to me after working with another medical practitioner who had recommended about twenty different vitamins and supplements. Patti noticed that after taking these supplements she had to go back on her asthma medication. When she came to the BioSET clinic, she had been on the medication for some time. I immediately tested her for the supplements and found she was sensitive to all but one of them. When she ceased taking them, she was able to discontinue her medication almost immediately, and she was free of symptoms for some time. This improvement occurred before she even began her BioSET clearings.

CREATING A SENSITIVITY MANAGEMENT PLAN

A sensitivity management plan defines the goals for getting asthma under control. These goals should include normal function of the airways and the ability to participate in physical or social activities without respiratory difficulty. They should also include sleeping through the night, no hospitalization, no emergency room visits or unscheduled visits to the physician, and no fear about what to do when breathing problems occur. The plan should incorporate a list of medications and why they are needed. Once a physician has approved of the plan, it should be kept in a place where it can be referred to often. Management plans may change as an asthmatic grows older, or according to changes in the environment, seasons, and so on. Eliminating and controlling sensitivities will also change the management plan. In formulating and adapting this plan, it is helpful for the BioSET practitioner to work in conjunction with a physician who specializes in asthma.

When developing their sensitivity management plan, an asthmatic should incorporate the answers to the following questions:

1. Do you already have an asthma allergy management plan?

2. Is it written down and do you understand it?

3. Do you know how to recognize and respond to an asthma episode?

4. Do you know how to recognize and respond to an asthma emergency?

5. Do you know what to do when recovering from an asthma or sensitivity episode?

6. When you are feeling better, should you keep taking medications?

7. Do you know how to keep an asthma episode from recurring?

Asthma sufferers need to educate themselves about sensitivity medications and the different kinds of asthma symptoms. These symptoms can be divided into noisy and quiet types. The noisy symptoms—wheezing, shortness of breath, tightness, and coughing—are easily recognized. The quiet symptom, compensatory breathing, is often not recognized as a precursor to the noisy symptoms. Often the body's compensation for breathing problems is so effective that the person does not realize the problem is a precursor to an asthma attack.

RECOGNIZING SYMPTOMS

Some people delay treating the quiet symptom, hoping it will go away. But immediate treatment can often prevent the onset of more serious symptoms. For this reason, it is important that asthmatics become attuned to changes in their breathing. A peak flow monitor is an inexpensive, handheld tool that measures the maximum speed with which air is forced out of the lungs. It can be invaluable for an asthmatic, since a reduced peak flow rate, which occurs when the bronchial tubes are blocked, may indicate a worsening condition. This instrument is particularly helpful with children who are not yet able to identify mild asthma symptoms. A stethoscope is also helpful for all asthmatics, but particularly for children, who can be taught to recognize abnormal breathing sounds by a physician or nurse. Recognizing symptoms makes early treatment with enzymes possible and may help a patient avoid the use of medications.

TAKING MEDICATIONS

Some asthmatics believe that taking a lot of medications will help cure them. But asthmatics should understand that medications only treat symptoms, they do not cure asthma. In any case, it is important to be aware of what each medication does. There are many types of drugs for asthma, including bronchodilators, cortical steroids, sedating and nonsedating antihistamines, decongestants, generic medications, prescription cough medicines, over-the-counter cough medicines, Tylenol, and aspirin. These can be delivered through inhalation, topical application, capsules, or sprinkling on food. Each asthmatic or parent of an asthmatic child should know how long each medication takes to work and the dosages appropriate for them and/or their children. They should know which are fast acting and which are long lasting, how often they should be used, and the best method of delivery. Delivery systems for asthma medication include metered dose inhalers, spacers, holding chambers, and nebulizers.

An inhaler, a canister that injects a medicated mist into a patient's airways, must be used properly, as instructed by a physician. A spacer is a hollow device added to an inhaler to extend the space between the metered dose inhaled and the patient's mouth. It coordinates the release of the medication and the timing of the slow aspiration to make sure the proper dose is received. This increases the medication's efficacy and makes sure it is deposited where it belongs. A nebulizer, commonly called a breathing machine, is designed to aerosolize medication into a fine mist of tiny particles and deliver those particles to the lungs. A nebulizer greatly improves the efficacy of medication delivery.

Asthmatics and parents of asthmatic children also need to know the purpose of each medication, how often it can be safely used in a twenty-four hour period, and what alternatives are available. For example, if they notice the quiet symptom, compensatory breathing, can they use enzymes and acupressure instead? This information should be written down in the management plan. Asthmatics should also be checked to make sure they are not sensitive to their medications, and, if they are, they should be cleared for those medications, if possible by a BioSET practitioner (visit www.bioset.net for referrals in your area).

In many cases, sensitivity proofing or otherwise altering their environment, changing their diet to eliminate food allergens, and eating only hormone-free, pesticide-free meat will be enough to allow an asthmatic to discontinue medications even before much sensitivity clearing work is done. The more responsibility people take for their own health, the fewer medications they will need, which is why a self-management plan is so important.

To take more responsibility for their condition, an asthmatic should take the following list of questions to ask their physicians about the medications they are taking:

+ What is the name of the medication and what is it supposed to do?
+ How long after I begin taking the medication will it have an effect?
+ When should I take it?
+ For how long should I take it?
+ How often should I take it?
+ What happens if the medication does not work?
+ Are there any foods, drinks, or other medications I should avoid while taking this medication?
+ Are there any side effects? If so, what should I do if they occur, and is there information available about them?

MANAGING WITH ALTERNATIVE THERAPIES

Asthma sufferers should try to manage their condition as much as possible with alternative therapies to avoid further stressing their immune systems with drug residues. They should have a good plan for avoiding episodes and maintaining a nonallergenic environment. Acupressure provides an alternative approach to early treatment. The diagram of acupressure points (see p. 153) shows points that can be stimulated for self-treatment. The lung points can be particularly helpful. There is also an area of the spine at C7 that asthmatics or people helping them can percuss (tap). This stimulation can help relieve asthma symptoms immediately.

Energetic techniques like qi-gong and breathing exercises can be helpful. Deep abdominal breathing is important. An asthmatic should avoid chest breathing as much as possible, inhaling and exhaling completely. Acupuncture, chiropractic, and spiritual practices that help provide an understanding of the emotions behind disease can also be helpful.

Homeopathy has several remedies for congestion, wheezing, and shortness of breath, including adrenalinum 6x, lobelia inflata 3x, belladonna 4x, ephedra vulgaris 4x, ipecacuanha 6x, solidago vigaurea 6x, and sambucus nigra 1x, though some people may be sensitive to these remedies. Adrenalinum is known for its ability to dilate or expand blood vessels and bronchial passages. Ipecacuanha is used for shortness of breath and constriction in the chest. Belladonna is used for tightness in the chest and labored breathing. Solidago vigaurea helps to eliminate heavy phlegm, coughing, and catarrh.

Experts talk about exercise-induced asthma, but I believe that many of those reactions are caused by sensitivities to hormones, adrenaline, and outdoor allergens. Once these are cleared, a patient may be able to exercise, enjoying activities such as bike riding, running, and walking. It is important to use discretion, though, and an asthmatic should never overexercise when unwell or suffering from an infection. Swimming may not be the best exercise for asthmatics, especially if they are sensitive to chlorine. And experts usually recommend activities that involve short bursts of energy rather than exercise for an extended period of time.

Ginkgo is a traditional herb in Chinese medicine that can be helpful for asthmatics. The biologically active compounds occur primarily in the leaves of the ginkgo tree and are classified as ginkgo-flavoneglycosides and terpenoids. The terpenoids have been demonstrated in a multitude of research to increase circulation and reduce the inflammatory response.

As asthmatics go through BioSET clearings, there will be less need for medications or alternative therapies for threatened attacks. It is important to consult with a physician and adjust medications as your need for them begins to lesson.

Breast-Feeding

Breast-feeding a baby for at least one year can help prevent the development of food sensitivities. If the mother does not breast-feed, the child should be put on a milk-free formula.

A mother who is breast-feeding should use digestive enzymes and be prudent about eating large amounts of common allergens because these allergens can be passed on to her child. Children should not be introduced to foods that are common allergens, including dairy, wheat, nuts, and other foods discussed in the food sensitivity section, until they are at least a year old. Foods that have caused problems for the mother in the past should be avoided during breast-feeding. When children start eating solid food, foods should be introduced one at a time to see whether the child shows a sensitivity to any of them. Muscle testing can help to determine this as well.

The Adolescent and Asthma

Taking responsibility and doing what is needed for an asthmatic condition can be particularly difficult for an adolescent. Having an adolescent daughter, I know that it is sometimes hard to communicate effectively with them, but it is essential that they realize they have a potentially life-threatening condition that must be monitored. Because most adolescents feel a need to assert their independence from their parents and are particularly sensitive to the influence of their peers, they may resist or ignore suggestions from their parents or their physician.

However, adolescent asthmatics must participate in their own health care. They need to be educated about their condition, how to treat it, and how to manage it to prevent symptoms from occurring. They need to know about nutrition, digestion, and the importance of eating good food to stay healthy. BioSET can be particularly helpful for adolescents because it can reduce the number of allergens they need to avoid and make managing their asthma relatively carefree instead of overwhelming.

Adolescence, like other periods of life, has its stresses, peer pressures, sense of competition, and the temptations to indulge in drugs, alcohol, and tobacco. The recent increase in teen smoking is a serious problem, and teenage asthmatics need to understand how damaging smoking or being around smoke can be for them. It has been reported that more than 90 percent of new tobacco users are children, and each day an estimated three thousand youths, ranging in age from ten to sixteen, begin to smoke for the first time.[1] Studies have shown that three-fourths of youths who use cigarettes continue to do so because they find it hard to quit. They may even end up as lifetime users. President Clinton signed a bill in August 1996 that was designed to prevent the sale of tobacco to underage users.

Not only the tobacco, but the chemicals in cigarettes, such as tar, nicotine, carbon monoxide, formaldehyde, aluminum, sulfur, and lead, have all been shown to cause health problems and to irritate and inflame the airways of people with asthma. Exposure to these toxins, whether by smoking or by being around secondhand smoke, can trigger severe asthmatic attacks.

Remove Allergens and Sensitivities from the Environment

No machine will remove particles and cigarette smoke. If guests or family members must smoke, having them smoke outside is the most reliable solution. Ventilation is key, and the EPA says that opening windows can be helpful, as indoor air may be more polluted than outdoor air.

Keeping indoor humidity below 50 percent can help to reduce dust mites and mold. Even better, one of the best ways to reduce house dust mites is to get rid of carpeting and use hard-floor surfacing instead. Vacuuming every day with a machine that has a HEPA (high-efficiency particulate arresting) filter and dusting with a duster that uses an electrostatic cloth will help reduce dust.

AIR-CONDITIONING AND FANS

Central air-conditioning is the most effective way of controlling humidity, though some people react to the cooler air. Air-conditioning vent openings are prime locations for the buildup of molds and so should be cleaned often. Window fans can draw pollens and molds into a house, and swamp coolers should be avoided because they can increase humidity.

AIR CLEANERS

Air cleaners, or air filters, are devices that filter the air in the home to remove airborne allergens. They can be invaluable for asthmatics. Several filtering devices are available, and some can be used in conjunction with forced-air cooling and heating systems. One type of filter uses standard disposable fiberglass filters that need to be changed monthly. Permanent air filters with baffles should be cleaned periodically. A third alternative, an electric filter that uses an electrostatic precipitator, requires frequent cleaning and can produce irritating ozone if not well maintained. The most effective filter is a HEPA filter.

Among the many things to consider when picking out an air filter is the amount of air the unit can circulate and clean. There are various advantages and disadvantages to the mechanical and electrical methods of air filtering. A mechanical filtration system can become more efficient with use and does not produce ozone, but it can only be used in homes that have forced-air heating and cooling systems. They also require frequent cleaning and can become coated with tars from tobacco smoke and lose their static charge capability. An ion generator, which has a very low electrical operating cost, does not require filter replacement for basic models. The disadvantages are that they can produce ozone, create iron imbalance in room air, and cause cleaning problems when air particles stick to the walls and furniture.

The FDA only lists a few air cleaners as medical devices. While the agency has not established performance standards, the machines listed in appendix B are probably all valuable health care products. Only one kind of purifier, however, is used in the environment where human life, health, and safety are most at risk—the operating room—and those are HEPA filtration systems. HEPA filtration systems require no maintenance, and their efficacy increases with use. An air cleaner that uses a true HEPA filter is the most efficient and reliable method of cleaning the air. If you wish to purchase a quality air filter, visit www.realgoods.com.

PORTABLE AIR CLEANERS

Concerns about indoor air quality and the rising incidence of asthma have made air cleaners a big business. Are air cleaners truly necessary? And can they remove enough dust, pollen, tobacco smoke, pet dander, microbes, and toxic outgassing? It depends upon the air cleaner and the amount of indoor pollution. The Environmental Protection Agency (EPA) and the American Lung Association do not recommend depending upon air cleaners as a first line of defense against allergens.

If a person does decide to buy an air cleaner, selecting one is quite a task. The problem is that there is no standard. The Association of House Appliance Manufacturers (AHAM) and the Consumers' Union (publisher of *Consumers Reports*) have different ways of evaluating air cleaners. Nevertheless, asthmatics *have* reported improvements when using air cleaners in their homes. Unfortunately, few air filters have been tested in placebo-controlled clinical studies that show their effect on people with asthma and sensitivities. More information on air filters can be found in appendix B.

VACUUM CLEANERS

Vacuum cleaners are another important piece of equipment for asthmatics. It is important to know whether your vacuum really eliminates dirt and dust from your home or merely recycles tiny particles back into the air, which is what most vacuums do. These particles can linger in the air for up to an hour, where they may continue to provoke sensitivity and asthmatic reactions.

Since many varieties of vacuums are available, I suggest that people do some research on them. Vacuum cleaners with HEPA filters can trap particles as small as .3 microns. Considering that a hair is between 75 and 100 microns thick and a dust mite is approximately 5 microns, .3 microns is tiny indeed; in fact, it is smaller than many of the particles that are breathed into the lungs. These vacuums can be extremely expensive, however. Vacuums that use a water filter are less expensive, and many asthmatics have found them useful. Allergy control filters can also be added to some canister vacuums.

HEAT SOURCES

For asthmatics, electric and hot-water radiant heaters are the best heating choices. Forced air can disperse dust and mold, and even if there is a central filter, ducts can accumulate large amounts of dust and mold. If forced air is used, the ducts should be cleaned once a year, and bedroom air vents should be closed to keep allergens from other parts of the home out of the bedroom of the family member with asthma. Fireplaces and wood-burning stoves are not recommended sources of heat because they can emit toxic particles and gases that cause respiratory problems. Kerosene heaters can produce sulfur dioxide and carbon monoxide in the home, which can be triggers for asthma.

WATER FILTERS

Pollutants, such as insecticides, fungicides, herbicides, fumigants, and other harmful chemicals, can leak into the public water supply. For this reason, I suggest to all my clients that they and their children drink either bottled spring water or filtered water, as opposed to tap water. Purchasing a water filter is one of the most important things you can do for your family.

Take Control of Your Home Environment

Having a healthy, sensitivity-free home environment is crucial to one's quality of life. Below are room- and allergen-specific tips for achieving this goal.

THE BEDROOM

It is particularly important to clear the sleeping environment of allergens because symptoms tend to worsen at night and may cause an asthmatic to wake up with an asthma attack. Several factors have been implicated in this characteristic pattern. Irritation from food or acid reflux can be a cause of asthma at night, as can allergens such as house dust and molds that are more active at night. Allergens inhaled earlier in the day may cause delayed reactions when the body is less active, and certain chemical mediators and hormones in the body that are known to affect asthma tend to rise or fall during the night. For example, histamine levels go up at night while adrenaline and steroid levels fall. This fluctuation can help to trigger a sensitivity response or attack. Everyone's lungs, even those of nonasthma sufferers, tend to constrict slightly in the evening hours. When the sun comes up, the body relaxes and the airways open up.

Allergens in the bedroom can be reduced by removing mold, down comforters, feather pillows, and the foam and kapok in mattresses and cushions. Asthmatics and allergy sufferers also should check their bed for possible allergens. Fabrics, detergents, and chlorine bleaches are possible irritants. For this reason, asthmatics should find a detergent that is not irritating to them and stick to it. Clothes should be rinsed twice to thoroughly eliminate any detergent residues.

BioSET practitioners clear patients for common allergens in the bedroom air. First, the person is asked to leave an open jar of water in their bedroom for twenty-four hours. Then they are cleared for whatever substances are suspended in the water. This technique clears for various gases that may be given off in the bedroom by furniture, fabrics, carpets, and other items that might be difficult to identify individually. The person is also tested and cleared for sensitivities to materials commonly used in bedding, including wool, acrylic, nylon, polyester, and cotton.

I worked with one young boy who snored regularly and woke up each morning with congestion. I treated him for foods and many environmental allergens, but nothing helped with the snoring. His mother mentioned that he might be sensitive to his polyester blanket. Sure enough, when I cleared him for polyester, he stopped snoring and no longer had congestion. It was an incredible overnight change.

I once knew a man who was very sensitive to electricity. He had severe problems with asthma until he worked with several doctors and realized that the electricity surrounding his bed was causing his problem. This electricity included clocks, lights, and other electrical devices. When I cleared him for electricity, his asthma completely disappeared.

Animals in the bedroom may have left behind their urine, saliva, and hair. Wallpaper, paint, books that collect dust, fabrics, wood floors, and rugs can also cause problems. One asthmatic told me that she was bothered by the natural floral scent in a potpourri near her bed. When she removed the potpourri, her wheezing and chest tightness subsided.

Since dust mites are one of the most common allergens that trigger asthmatics, it is important to get rid of accumulations of dust. Clearing for dust with BioSET is usually effective, but until that is done many steps can be taken to clean the indoor environment. There should be smooth, uncluttered surfaces in the bedroom, with few small objects like books, knickknacks, CDs, tapes, or stuffed animals. All of these should be put in drawers if possible. Bedrooms should not be used as libraries or studies. Bedding should be washed weekly in hot water—135 degrees Fahrenheit—to kill dust mites. Cool water just gives them a bath. Pillows can be encased in nonallergic and nonpermeable dust-proof covers, if the person sleeping on them is not sensitive to the material. Otherwise, the cover will do more harm than good. Avoid feather comforters and pillows, and remove carpeting if possible. Carpeting is a major hiding place for dust mites.

Avoid wall pennants, macramé hangings, and other dust catchers. Stuffed toys should be machine washable. Keep all clothing in a closet with the door closed. When vacuuming or dusting, be sure to use a dust face mask.

THE KITCHEN

In the kitchen, exhaust fans can remove water vapor during cooking. Mold grows in refrigerators, particularly around door gaskets, in water pans below self-defrosting refrigerators, and on spoiled foods. Mold can also grow on garbage, so containers should be emptied and cleaned frequently.

THE BATHROOM

In the bathroom, excess water should be removed from shower doors, tiles, and tubs with a squeegee. Shower curtains, bath tile, shower stalls, tubs, and toilet tanks should all be washed with mold-preventive solutions. Do not carpet the bathroom.

CHLORINE

The effects of chlorine, a common sensitivity for asthmatics, are particularly noticeable after a shower. There may be difficulty breathing and a feeling of running out of oxygen. Some asthmatics have found that a chlorine-removing filter on the showerhead helps to prevent this reaction. BioSET treatment is also recommended, however, since a filter cannot eliminate all the chlorine.

TOILETRIES

Asthma attacks can also be caused by chemicals found in certain types of creams, sunscreens, and soaps. There are eight thousand known chemicals found in common toiletries, many of which have not been tested by the FDA. Perfumes and cosmetics derived from petroleum and coal tar can be as bad as cigarette smoke for asthmatics. The scent contained in perfumes, lotions, soaps, cosmetics, detergents, and other products can cause migraine, dizziness, rashes, and eczema.

Learning about and using natural soaps and skin care products—as well as natural house-cleaning products—can make a huge and immediate difference in respiratory health and allergy symptoms.

Until these sensitivities are cleared with BioSET, it is important to employ an air purifier whenever possible and to use fragrance-free products.

LAUNDRY ROOMS AND BASEMENTS

In the laundry room, vent the dryer outside and dry clothing immediately after washing. In a basement, do not lay carpet and pads on a concrete floor. Use vinyl flooring instead. Dirt floors should be covered with a vapor barrier. Keep the basement free of dust, and remove stored items that are likely to harbor mold. Sensitive individuals should not have their bedroom on a basement level.

PAINTING AND REMODELING

Painting and remodeling a house can be toxic for anyone, and particularly for an asthmatic. All the materials used and the gases they emit are possible asthma triggers. I test and clear people for latex, oil, and acrylic-based paints, as well as for glues, hardwoods, and hardwood finishes. Until these clearings can be done, asthmatics should avoid these products.

HOUSEHOLD PETS

Approximately 10 percent of the American population, including 20–30 percent of asthmatics, are sensitive to animals. Most have a sensitivity to cats, which is actually a sensitivity to dander and the proteins in their saliva and urine. It is estimated that 70 percent of the homes in the United States have at least one cat or dog.[2] Approximately six million Americans are sensitive to cats, and early exposure can lead to asthma in a child with a predisposition. Keeping an animal outdoors is preferable, but that also can create a problem because outdoor allergens—pollen and mold—can cling to the fur and come off when the animal is touched.

Frequent bathing of a cat is important, as is appropriate indoor and outdoor ventilation and frequent vacuuming with a HEPA filter vacuum cleaner. Cat allergen can linger in carpets, mattresses, and walls for months and even years. To speed up removal, clean heating and air-conditioning ducts thoroughly, clean the walls, have carpets and upholstery professionally cleaned, and use HEPA air cleaners throughout the house.

Studies have shown that washing a cat with water removes much of its surface sensitivity content and reduces the future production of allergens. Place the cat or kitten in the sink and pour lukewarm water over its body. Wash it weekly for three weeks, then at two- or three-week intervals after that. An asthmatic should wear a face mask when brushing a cat, and then wash their hands and change their clothes after touching it—another reminder that parasites can be picked up while touching an animal. Since small animals like mice and gerbils also bear allergens, wear a mask when cleaning their cage or have a nonsensitive person do it.

Beware Other Problem Areas Indoors

Antique shops can harbor a lot of mold, as can sleeping bags, greenhouses, summer cottages, hotel rooms, and automobile air conditioners. Farmers, gardeners, bakers, upholsterers, paperhangers, millworkers, florists, food preparers, plumbers, librarians, and people working around moldy materials all have occupational exposure to mold.

Two other highly toxic environments are hair and nail salons, which can be hazardous to anyone with respiratory problems. Many of the chemicals used in nail care are common allergens, especially acetone, which is used in nail polish remover and hair chemicals.

Be Well Outdoors

If you suffer from asthma, avoid cutting grass or raking leaves, or use a well-fitted mask while doing so. Avoid exposure to soil, compost, sandboxes, hay, and fertilizers. Correct drainage problems near the house to get rid of any pooled water. Avoid camping or walking in the woods where mold grows around logs or other vegetation. Remove rotted logs from around the house and yard.

Air pollution can also worsen asthma by irritating the lungs. Small particles in the air due to vehicles and industrial plants, along with ground-level ozone, get into the lungs and cause an inflammatory reaction. Ground-level ozone is especially problematic during the summer, when sunlight reacts with fuel emissions to produce high levels of ozone, particularly in urban areas. Ozone exposure has been shown to correlate with chest pain, difficulty breathing, and reduced lung function.[3]

What should people do? To cut down on ozone pollution, asthmatics and people in general are urged to reduce vehicle trips and engine idling, limit the use of gasoline-powered lawn and garden equipment, and conserve energy, such as setting air conditioners to higher temperatures. Air quality is paramount. A BioSET clearing for ozone can be done at home. Simply place a container of water outdoors for an hour (or even in your car) to collect air. This clearing will probably need to be done periodically for relief.

Maintain Healthy Car Environments

Many people are sensitive to substances in their car environment, including fuel, exhaust fumes, plastics, hydrocarbons, carpets, and synthetic leathers. Someone I know had excruciating back pain whenever she sat on the synthetic leather seats in my car. An air purifier can help in the car, but there is no way to escape from fuel or exhaust fumes or to effectively avoid contact with interior materials. These sensitivities should be cleared with BioSET.

Manage Diseases

Certain diseases can trigger asthmatic responses. It is important to watch for the spread of certain viruses.

INFLUENZA

When an asthmatic is exposed to a flu or cold virus, there is a high risk of developing symptoms that can trigger asthma. To prevent the spread of viruses, cover your mouth when sneezing or coughing, wash your hands frequently, dispose of used tissues, and keep your hands away from your face. Viruses spread from person to person through the air from coughs and sneezes, through hand contact with an infected person, or by touching surfaces that have been contaminated and then rubbing the eyes, mouth, or nose.

CHICKEN POX

Chicken pox (varicella) is a relatively harmless childhood illness, but it can be troublesome for an asthmatic. Children who have been treated with cortical steroids may be at particular risk because these steroids suppress the immune system, which can lead to serious complications from chicken pox, even death. The symptoms of chicken pox include a rash, with tiny, clear red-based blisters, accompanied by a fever. Once a child who is receiving oral or injected cortical steroids is exposed to the virus, a physician should be notified immediately. The child can be treated within forty-eight hours after exposure with an injection of varicella immune globulin, an antibody preparation. I also find it helpful to clear with BioSET for the chicken pox virus.

Enjoy Massage and Chiropractic Care

Another preventive measure that has been proven to be effective with asthmatics is massage. Research has indicated that a weekly upper-body massage may help asthmatics find relief from symptoms such as chest tightness, wheezing, and fatigue. In one study, asthmatics who received weekly fifteen-minute upper-body massages reported drops in chest tightness, wheezing, physical pain, and fatigue. Even with the best results, massage will not prevent asthmatics from having to take medication, but the results have led people to realize that stress plays a major role in asthma.

Stress plays a major role in any chronic illness. In an emotional situation asthmatics will often feel an immediate tightness in the chest and have difficulty breathing. No matter how much stress they are under, however, if the body is free of allergens and in a state of homeostasis and digestion is good, I believe they will be strong enough to deal with any emotional situation without experiencing an asthma attack. A balanced chemistry, good digestion, and a strong immune system are necessary for asthmatics to deal with the stresses that are common to the society in which we live.

PART THREE

BioSET
(Bioenergetic Sensitivity and Enzyme Therapy)

Defining BioSET

BioSET (Bioenergetic Sensitivity and Enzyme Therapy) is a natural holistic health care system based on energetic medicine and meridian therapy that works to prevent and resolve chronic health conditions such as asthma and sinusitis. BioSET is comprised of three branches of healing:

* Enzyme therapy, including nutrition and proper diet
* Organ-specific detoxification
* A revolutionary, noninvasive, and usually permanent technique for eliminating food and environmental sensitivities

A Brief History of BioSET

The BioSET system emerged from my broad experience with sensitivity therapies in clinical practice, drawing on a body of knowledge gained from other health care professionals as well as from patients. It also reflects my own desire for healing and personal growth, which began as I searched for a therapy that would clear my own food sensitivities. In the years that took me from chiropractic college to medical school and through my postgraduate education, I examined and evaluated every available treatment, finally concentrating on enzyme therapy, which I discuss in *MicroMiracles: Discover the Healing Power of Enzymes* (Rodale, 2005). As I began to take digestive enzymes myself, I was surprised to notice relief from many of my symptoms, although some foods still left me feeling tired or depressed. As my practice grew over time, I was able to explore other therapeutic possibilities, including procedures and products that could ease the food sensitivities my patients and I shared.

I developed the BioSET system over twenty-five years of clinical practice and study, and it offers anyone the opportunity to achieve and maintain a healthy lifestyle. Integrating traditional Chinese medicine and acupressure with a contemporary understanding of applied immunology and nutrition, the BioSET system is simple and easy to use. Although complex cases should be treated by a trained practitioner, anyone can learn some forms of acupressure, fingertip stimulation of points on the body, for use in home sensitivity treatments.

Applied gently and correctly, acupressure can have a beneficial impact on the immune system as well as on many other body systems. Traditional Chinese medicine refers to the most important pressure points located along both sides of the spine as "association points," suggesting the association between the locations and the energy flowing through the body. Through massage, these points are stimulated to reprogram the body's sensitivites. Because these association points are readily accessible, a patient can remain completely clothed during this treatment.

Diagnostic Procedures and Treatments

There are two ways that BioSET practitioners can measure the body's vital energy to discover whether it is balanced—the ideal state of health—or whether it has become weakened or stressed. The first is muscle testing, which I will discuss in chapter 10. The second is by way of an EAV, the electronic device described in chapter 2, which is calibrated to accurately measure the flow of a body's energy meridians.

A BioSET practitioner then assesses the need for the following treatments:

+ Specific digestive enzymes and systemic enzymes (supplements that use nutrients and botanicals to balance organs, tissues, and cells)

+ Homeopathic drops for organ-specific detoxification and drainage

+ BioSET desensitization, an acupressure technique that utilizes allergen frequencies and energetics to fully clear and/or reprogram a patient, via the nervous and meridian systems, of any allergen or sensitivity. BioSET balances meridians that allergens have blocked, which have produced a multiplicity of health symptoms that may have become chronic. This natural noninvasive desensitization can clear most sensitivities almost permanently.

BioSET practitioners also employ kinesiology, acupuncture, and chiropractic diagnostic tools to help diagnose blockages and remove them. Restoring the flow of vital energies through the meridians is essential since particular blockages correspond to specific reactions to sensitivities, such as asthma symptoms.

The BioSET technique can be practiced by any health practitioner, including doctors, nurses, acupuncturists, chiropractors, dentists, and, to some extent, clients themselves, including those who suffer from asthma. Clinical studies with BioSET have demonstrated that it is by far the most successful and succinct treatment for the elimination of sensitivities.

BioSET Works with Electromagnetic Energy

BioSET is based on a theory that views the body as being made up of pathways that allow the flow of electromagnetic energy. In *The Energy Within: The Science Behind Every Oriental Therapy from Acupuncture to Yoga*, Richard M. Chin, MD, OMD, refers to the body as "a matrix of interacting multidimensional energy fields." He writes that every person has an inner energy flowing through his or her mind and body that is a reflection of universal energies. When these energies are out of balance or stop flowing, we experience illness or disease. Keeping our energy moving and in balance can prevent illness and create a maximum state of health.

According to Chin, there are three types of energy:

+ Genetic or prenatal energy, which is the energy level to which a person is genetically disposed. It is programmed in the genes like the color of a person's eyes and hair, height, and so on.

+ Core energy, which is a combination of the energy a person is born with and the energy that forms their body. It is a combination of two prenatal energies.

+ Acquired energy, which is the energy a person acquires during their lifetime via their lifestyle and practices. This type of energy is within an individual's control.

The genetic or prenatal energy, known as qi (sometimes spelled chi) in Chinese, is thought to be the source and the destination of all creation. Qi must keep moving in order to sustain life. In order for energy to move, it must have an inherent polarity relationship, which means it must have somewhere to go. Eastern practitioners—who look at the body from a holistic perspective that considers the energy imbalances of the entire system, rather than simply the disease of a particular organ or body part—have discovered a highly organized system of energy channels or pathways, another circulatory system similar to the cardiovascular and nervous systems. This is the system that transports qi.

Chin writes:

> Governed by yin and yang, sometimes described as positive and negative charges, our energy flows along very specific but invisible channels or pathways throughout our bodies. This complex network forms a veritable energy 'road map.' But these 'lines of energy' are actually just the centers of many three-dimensional fields that together comprise our internal energy system and our external aura, much like the energy fields surrounding magnets.
>
> Pain or illness results when the flow of energy becomes blocked or unbalanced in some way, because this disharmony then upsets the balance of the body's entire energy system. . . Although some energetic healing techniques engage the entire system, many only need to work with the body's twelve primary channels and two governing vessels (channels that oversee all others) to create complete balance and health. One method of balancing the body's energy system is acupuncture, which uses tiny needles to stimulate specific points along the twelve primary energy channels and two governing vessels.
>
> Each of the twelve primary channels in this corresponds to one of the body's twelve primary energetic organs. In energetic medicine, an organ, too, is actually an energy system that can only be understood in its relationship to the body's entire energy system.

TWELVE PRIMARY CHANNELS AND TWO GOVERNING VESSELS

The concept of twelve primary channels and two governing vessels is important to understanding how BioSET works. An initial clearing with BioSET evaluates blockages in a body's energy channels in relationship to specific allergens.

The first channel is the lung channel, which regulates the body's entire energy system and oversees the intake of oxygen. Disharmony in this channel is experienced as coughing, asthma, sensitivities, skin problems, bronchitis, and fatigue.

The second channel is the large intestine channel, which regulates the body's waste removal activities. Disharmony here could result in a distended abdomen, constipation, and diarrhea.

The third channel is the stomach channel, which regulates the body's ability to take in food and fluids. Disharmony here may lead to mouth sores, nausea, and vomiting.

The fourth channel is the spleen channel, which regulates the transformation of food into energy and the maintenance of blood supply. Disharmony could result in poor appetite, anemia, menstrual problems, chronic hepatitis, and fatigue.

The fifth channel is the heart channel, which rules the head and houses the spirit. It regulates the blood vessels. Disharmony or unbalanced flow here may lead to heart palpitations or insomnia.

The sixth channel is the small intestines channel, which draws out energy from food and leaves the remains as waste. Disharmony may result in vomiting or abdominal pain.

The seventh channel is the bladder, which receives and excretes urine fluid waste. Disharmony could result in burning sensations when urinating or in incontinence.

The eighth channel is the kidney channel, which stores reproductive energy and oversees maintenance of bones. Disharmony can result in backaches, chronic ear problems, and chronic asthma.

The ninth channel is the pericardium channel, which protects and oversees the heart channel. Disharmony can result in stress, chest tightening sensations, and a variety of breathing problems.

The tenth channel is the triple burner, which oversees the body's water processing, retaining what is needed and excreting the rest. Disharmony may be experienced as edema, a stiff neck, or water retention.

The eleventh channel is the gallbladder, which stores and secretes bile, a fluid that helps transforms food into energy. Disharmony may be experienced as a bitter taste in one's mouth, nausea, and jaundice.

The twelfth channel is the liver channel, which regulates the entire energy system and oversees maintenance of blood supplies. Disharmony may lead to high blood pressure, dizziness, PMS, muscle spasms, and eye problems.

Of the remaining two channels, the thirteenth is the governing vessel, and the fourteenth is the conception vessel. They circulate energy through the other twelve channels.

FIVE BASIC QUALITIES OF ENERGY

There are five basic qualities of energy that need to be balanced within each channel. These respond to the five elements in Chinese practice and are called wood, fire, earth, metal, and water energy. If these energies are out of balance in any one channel, they can disrupt the delicate balance of the body's entire system.

MAPPING AND MEASURING ENERGY FLOW IN THE BODY

Studies have shown that the whole universe, from the tiniest atom to the largest galaxy, is controlled by electromagnetic forces. These forces are responsible for the shape of all things and govern their movement, inter-relationships, replication, and functions. This applies to stars, minerals, and atoms, as well as to all living things. The electromagnetic forces in the bodies of animals can be seen as lines of force that run near the surface of the body and then pass into deeper structures, which are the organs. These lines of force are called meridians, channels, or electromagnetic energy forces.

ACUPUNCTURE

The kind of energy that runs in the acupuncture meridians can be measured and recorded in the body's different organs. Acupuncture practitioners employ a variety of techniques to eliminate imbalances or blockages in the body's natural flow of energy. BioSET uses techniques drawn from acupuncture and acupressure, medical immunology, and kinesiology to do just this—locate and remove blockages in electromagnetic pathways that are related to allergens, as well as to digestive stress and toxicity.

GALVANIC SKIN RESPONSE

Several areas of scientific study have given indications of how these energy systems in the body operate and can be detected. Studies of galvanic skin response, for example—the bodily response that lie detectors measure—have provided interesting data. Another study found the presence of an organized system of highly electroconductive points on the skin, similar to the system of points used for centuries in traditional Chinese medicine.[1] These points are related to the human autonomic nerve reflexes, and irregularities in the points correlate with clinical medical diagnoses. Using a new technique, scientists are now able to use photography to locate and identify those points.

Neurophysicists have known for a long time that when they measure the galvanic skin response (GSR) at different points on a person's skin, it varies in direct relation to the amount of energy being discharged from the autonomic nervous system. Decreased electrical resistance at certain points on the skin is influenced by autonomic sweat gland activity on the skin's surface, by the concentrations of nerve fibers beneath the skin, and by muscle motor points. This means that any physical disorder that intensifies autonomic activity will decrease electrical resistance on those areas of the skin related to the autonomic nervous system.

Skin resistance has been measured in the laboratory by having a person hold one electrode and passing the other over their skin. As early as 1950, one researcher, Y. Nakatani, proposed a system of electrodiagnosis and electrotreatment that was based on correlations he had found between differences in skin resistance at certain points on the skin and physical illness. His system, which is called Ryodoraku, is based on the fact that one of the ways internal disease manifests itself is by causing a disturbance in the autonomic nervous system. The disturbance may be manifested systematically by increased nerve response at certain points.

Nakatani found that internal disturbances could be detected, often before they manifested clinically, by measuring skin resistance. Nakatani also noticed that anatomical locations of electroconductive points in unhealthy subjects varied with the disease. Subjects with the same disease had most of their points in the same location. All of these electroconductive points were remarkably close in location and about equal to the number of points found in Oriental acupuncture charts of the human body. Nakatani used electrical stimulation to normalize highly conductive points.

KIRLIAN PHOTOGRAPHY

B. K. Kirlian developed another approach to studying this phenomenon in 1961. He devised a method for photographing the electromagnetic discharges emanating from various objects. This Kirlian phenomena and its possible relationship to electroconductive body points triggered much new research on the topic. Researchers wondered if the Kirlian effect was a result of discharges coming from galvanically detectable electroconductive skin points.

Kirlian photography is a good illustration of electromagnetic forces in the body. Perhaps visual and photographic analysis of these electroconductive points can assist in detecting and diagnosing diseases that have not yet manifested clinically.

SENDING NEW MESSAGES TO THE BRAIN

The interesting thing about traditional Chinese medicine, studies of galvanic skin response, and Kirlian photography is that they all produce evidence of a pattern of electromagnetic points on the skin—and all the patterns look more or less the same. We know that these points are related to underlying autonomic nerve activity and that they respond to stimulation by electricity, needles, heat, and pressure.

Researchers who have tested traditional acupuncture meridians to see whether they are direct current paths have found that these meridians conduct electricity toward the spinal cord. The researchers concluded that the meridians carry messages to the brain, which responds by sending back the electrical current needed to stimulate healing. This concept also helps explain how BioSET clearings work. We stimulate the nervous system to send new messages to the brain.

THE CHAKRAS

In addition to the acupuncture meridians, many systems identify seven energy centers, called chakras, which are located in the body along the spine. There are two contradictory views that attempt to explain the body's electromagnetic structure and the chakras. The first is that biological structures produce the electromagnetic field in the body. In this view, electrochemical activity within nerve plexi is thought to create the energy vortexes called chakras. The body is thought to produce an electrical current that is transformed and processed by boosters—the acupuncture points—and carried by power circuits—the acupuncture meridians.

The opposite view is that the electromagnetic energy produces the physical body. In this view, order begins to emerge from random activity in the quantum realm, replicates itself, and becomes a pattern. More precise patterns develop until a physical form emerges from information and energy is carried on an electromagnetic wave. Before it becomes physical, the body's energy pattern is an aura, or what biologist Rupert Sheldrake calls a morphogenic field. The role of the chakras, according to this theory, may be to process information carried on particular frequencies.

CHIROPRACTIC AND THE HUMAN ENERGY FIELD

The whole concept of the body as an energy field was not new to me when I learned BioSET. As a chiropractic student, I was introduced to a philosophy that regards the body as more than just matter, muscles, and tissues coming together without any real intelligence. Chiropractic acknowledges that the body is a holistic complex and that the universal or innate intelligence or organizing force that pervades the vast galaxies also pervades the simplest cells of the body. The founder of chiropractic, Dr. D. D. Palmer, talked about the concept of electromagnetic energy fields. He said that the mind does not control the functions of the body. Instead, there is an innate intelligence that controls the mind and its functions as well as the functions of the body. This innate intelligence has the power to conceive, judge, and reason about matters pertaining to the body's internal welfare. The healing art of chiropractic has been around for one hundred years, during which time it has been successfully treating the body while appreciating it as more than matter.

In the chiropractic view, when a bone is out of alignment or the spine is distorted or misaligned, the energy force in the body is cut off, and this in turn can cause serious disease. When the misalignments or imbalances are corrected, the energy can flow again through the nervous system to the brain, and homeostasis is restored.

How Energy Blockages Cause Health Problems

Any time there are energy blockages in the body, health problems of some sort inevitably result. Some areas of the body are weaker for genetic reasons. Therefore, they will have the greatest reaction to allergens, weakening other areas of the body as well. Common symptoms produced by such blockages include aches and pains, sore throat, fever, chills, painful lymph nodes, weakness, extreme fatigue, headaches, sleep disturbances, irritability, confusion, depression, forgetfulness, a burning sensation somewhere in the body, frequent urination, sores in the mouth, indigestion, bloating, water retention, and even extreme emotional responses such as crying spells or suicidal behavior. After working with BioSET for twenty-five years, I have to conclude that most health problems have their roots in some type of response to allergens.

If blockages continue or a body is constantly exposed to a sensitivity, the blockages can spread throughout the system, causing more serious problems. When the immune system becomes overloaded and compromised trying to deal with all of these problems, autoimmune problems can develop. Over time, as it is bombarded with sensitivities, a body becomes more susceptible to chronic health problems and decreased energy levels. In extreme circumstances, migraines, tumors, and mental problems might result.

CLEARING MERIDIANS

BioSET uses acupressure techniques to stimulate the areas of the body that are connected to blockages in a person's energy system. If a blockage affects a certain organ, the practitioner stimulates areas of the nervous system connected to that organ by automatic nerve impulses. For example, a sensitivity to dairy products might affect the reproductive organs or cause a blockage in the reproductive meridian. To treat for a dairy sensitivity, a practitioner would stimulate areas of the nervous system related to the reproductive system. By stimulating those areas, which are located along the spine, while a person is holding the allergen in their hand, the electromagnetic repulsion to that allergen is eliminated and a chemical or enzymatic change occurs, neutralizing the immune mediators and interrupting the allergen or antigen-antibody complex reaction. This clears the energy blockage for the area involved and sends a message to the brain, stating that a person has been desensitized to dairy products. The body no longer identifies dairy as a sensitivity, and the energy blockages in response to dairy products no longer occur.

BioSET in Action

As mentioned earlier, BioSET employs three basic treatments: enzyme therapy, organ-specific detoxification, and desensitization.

UTILIZING ENZYMES

Enzymes make it possible for us to digest all the food we eat. The three types of enzymes—metabolic, digestive, and natural enzymes—play an important role in the biochemical reactions in our bodies, helping to deliver the nutrients in our digested food throughout our systems. Natural enzymes are present in the fruits and vegetables we eat, and the digestive enzymes responsible for breaking down those foods are secreted in the mouth, the stomach, the pancreas, and the small intestine. Unfortunately, our methods of preparing foods often destroy the natural enzymes in fruits and vegetables by canning, overcooking, or processing them for greater convenience.

We also often fail to chew our food well enough to let the digestive enzymes do their jobs. In our hurried lives, we have forgotten the pleasure of lingering over our food and enjoying its flavor, and as a result, we do not make the best use of the enzymes in our digestive systems. Few people chew their food the minimum of thirty times necessary to permit the proper work of digestive enzymes, not realizing that enzymes can be a natural cure for our digestive problems as well as for our food sensitivities. Chapter 13 provides an overview of the benefits of adding digestive enzymes to your diet.

DETOXIFYING AND PURIFYING YOUR BODY

The toxicity of our environment—both in our communities and in our homes—can have a dramatic impact on our health. In order to heal our sensitivities fully, we must be prepared to make changes to detoxify our living environments. This is especially important for asthmatics, who respond strongly to the toxicity of our industrial world. First, it is important to identify sources of toxic exposure and minimize contact with them (see chapter 8 for suggestions for detoxifying a home environment). Next, each person must take steps to clear toxins that have accumulated in their body by making detoxification part of their daily health practices.

A body's immune system is designed to prevent the invasion of microbes and tumor cells, but this protection can be compromised by poor digestion, toxicity, or inflammation caused by sensitivities. By clearing the toxins that accumulate in a body's cells and tissues, detoxification helps their immune system work efficiently and effectively, guarding vulnerable areas like the skin, lungs, and digestive tract. When an asthmatic successfully limits their exposure to toxic elements, they help their immune system defend against the threat of disease, so detoxification is key to beginning the natural healing process.

Drinking a generous amount of water each day helps to promote immediate detoxification. Juicing and fasting should be managed carefully, within a balanced nutritional plan that allows for regular cleansing of the digestive tract. Purification practices like breathing techniques, dry-skin brushing, and detoxifying baths and saunas are also beneficial. Homeopathic remedies and massage can often be useful and effective, as well.

CLEARING SENSITIVITIES

Desensitization treatment for asthmatics should always proceed with greater care when their sensitivities are severe. If a person's reactions place them at risk for shock (anaphylaxis), or if they have had a severe reaction in the past, it is important to work with a professional BioSET practitioner.

Sometimes what appears to be an allergic response can be a sign of a more serious underlying condition—a patient who reports nasal congestion on either the left or the right side, for example, may simply be responding to an allergen, but this type of congestion can also indicate the presence of a polyp, a tumor, or another health problem.

BioSET training prepares a practitioner to understand intricate problems, such as multiple food sensitivities (in which two or more foods together cause an allergic reaction) as well as sensitivities that implicate biochemistry and the regulation of hormones. A practitioner is also best suited to treat multiple chemical sensitivities, chronic fatigue syndrome, and environmental sensitivities. Most important, in the case of cross-reacting sensitivities, which involve the reactivity of specific acupoints or meridians, a practitioner's skill and experience are invaluable.

BioSET self-care (described in chapter 10) is not a substitute for treatment by an expert; in the same way, reading medical books can inform you about a condition without qualifying you to diagnose and treat it as a doctor. Please check the BioSET website at www.bioset.net for a list of qualified BioSET practitioners worldwide.

If a person has simple food sensitivities, they may respond well to self-care techniques. BioSET self-clearing works best for people who have identified their reactions to known sensitivities. If a scratch test or medical diagnosis has pointed to specific allergens, home care may be an appropriate way to clear their sensitivities, as long as their symptoms are mild to moderate, not severe or life threatening. A trained BioSET practitioner can offer guidance and support as they prepare to begin their home treatment, and most practitioners are open to the idea of having patients participate in self-care. A person can also review the procedures to check their technique by watching the video *Creating Wellness*, available from the BioSET Institute (see appendix B for more details).

At-Home Procedures: Muscle Testing and Clearings

If you do not have a BioSET practitioner in your area and wish to perform self-clearings at home, the easiest and most effective way to identify your sensitivities to environmental and food sensitivities is through a simple self-diagnostic procedure known as muscle testing. In order to accurately identify blockages and sensitivities, make sure to carefully follow the muscle testing procedures described in this book. This will be your primary and most crucial self-diagnostic tool, and your first step toward desensitization.

How Muscle Testing Works to Diagnose Imbalances

Quick and noninvasive, muscle testing offers a reliable means of locating the presence of a variety of problems—identifying sensitivities and nutritional imbalances, as well as pointing to structural misalignments in the body. It can even help to uncover physical problems arising from emotional issues.

This method identifies blockages in the electromagnetic energy fields when one is exposed to, or in contact with, an sensitivity, bypassing the conscious and subconscious minds. When a suspected sensitivity is held in the hand, a strong muscle will weaken if there is a sensitivity to the substance. A "strong" or "weak" muscle refers to the nervous system's response to the test, not to the literal strength of the muscle.

There are two types of muscle testing, O-ring testing and testing with a partner. If you have a friend or family member willing to help you with this, make sure that he or she reads the following directions carefully.

To prepare for this test, you will collect particular foods or environmental items that you wish to be tested against and put them into thin glass holders, such as wineglasses or vials (see appendix B for how to order these vials).

You and your partner will need to wash your hands prior to and between each test. If you don't wish to keep going into the kitchen or the bathroom, a damp cloth is sufficient. Since metals can interfere with a response, remove all watches, rings, and jewelry.

Place all of the test items at least four feet away from your body. To begin, you should sit comfortably in a chair, feet uncrossed and flat on the floor, while your partner stands on the opposite side of you from the arm being tested. For example, when testing your right arm, your partner should stand on your left side.

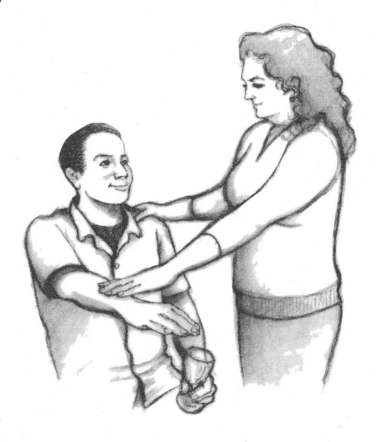

Your partner will ask you to raise your right arm at a ninety-degree angle in front of your body (pointing straight ahead of you). Your elbow should be straight, with the palm of your hand face down and your fingers pointing forward. Your partner will rest their right hand on your left shoulder and, with their left hand, make contact with your right arm just above the wrist. Your partner should then press gently downward with their left hand while asking you to resist against the downward pressure they are applying. This provides a base measure of how you naturally resist during a muscle test. Your partner will be able to compare your future responses to this strong example.

You are now ready to begin your sensitivity testing. Your partner will place a glass vial or a particular food in your left hand, the opposite hand from the arm being tested. Make sure that you hold a vial with your fingertips touching the place where the substance is in the glass. Next, your partner will push down on your outstretched right arm to see if your response remains strong. If you are sensitive to a particular item, you will be unable to hold your arm firmly against the testing force (your partner's gentle pressure), and your arm will collapse or weaken. If you are not sensitive to a particular food, your arm will not waver at all and your ability to lock against resistance will be evident. Any wavering in your right arm is a sign of a sensitivity.

It is important to remember that *your partner does not need to use great force when muscle testing*. To perform an effective muscle test, your partner needs only to be able to feel a clear difference between your "strong" and "weak" responses. When your partner asks you to resist their downward pressure, they will notice an immediate locking of the arm (a "strong" test) or a weakening and collapse (a "weak" test).

You may then proceed to test additional items for sensitivities. The average person will only be able to test for about ten items at any one sitting before their arm begins to tire, which would make testing inaccurate. However, you can double the number of tests at one time by switching to the other arm.

Note the substances to which you are sensitive on a chart, such as the following sample chart. This chart will be a guide for the clearings you will do.

BioSET Testing Chart

SUBSTANCE	CLEARED	SENSITIVITY REMAINS	OBSERVATIONS
Amino acids			
Phenolics			
Biochemicals			
Minerals			
Vitamin C			
B vitamins			
Sugars			
Vitamin A			
Vitamin E			
Vitamin D			
Fatty acids			
Additional foods			

I realized how easy and helpful muscle testing could be on one occasion, when my thirty-three-year-old friend Susan and I were walking to one of my book signings in Chicago. It was a lovely summer evening, and we stopped on the way to enjoy some delicious-looking fresh yellow cherries sold by a street vendor.

Only ten minutes later, Susan (a severe asthmatic) began to wheeze as we entered the bookstore. As the audience looked on, fascinated by this impromptu demonstration, I used the BioSET muscle testing technique to determine whether Susan was reacting to the cherries we had just eaten. Susan stretched out her right arm, while holding two cherries in her left hand. I pressed down on her right arm, which immediately weakened to indicate that she was very sensitive to the cherries. Performing the BioSET

Sensitivity Desensitization Technique as the audience watched, I treated Susan's sensitivity at once, and her wheezing stopped right away.

Self-Testing

If a partner is not available, you can test yourself using a form of muscle testing known as the O-ring test. You will make a circle by opposing your little finger and thumb on one hand. Then, with the index finger of the other hand, you will try to separate the two opposing fingers. Your fingers should be strong and inseparable. It they are not strong, there may be structural misalignment or carpal tunnel syndrome, which would render the technique ineffective.

If your circled fingers are strong when tugged on, the next step is to hold the substance or substance-filled vial in the hand being tested, or in the hand doing the testing, with your remaining three fingertips touching the substance or vial. If the two circled fingers remain strong when the index finger of the other hand pulls on them, you are not sensitive to the substance. If your circled fingers weaken and the circle separates, you are sensitive to the substance. This technique takes practice to learn, but it can be a survival tool for severely sensitive individuals who can use it to test their foods before eating.

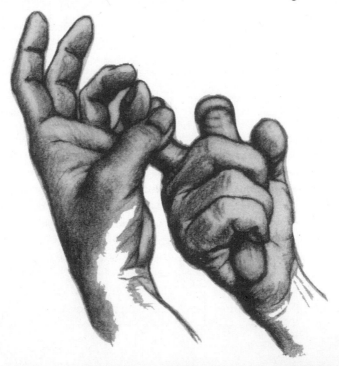

The BioSET Home Sensitivity-Clearing Procedure

Before I describe the BioSET at-home treatments, let me emphasize that their purpose is to desensitize a person to environmental and food allergens that they come in contact with every day, for example, a sensitivity to certain foods that seem to aggravate their asthma symptoms. This home treatment is *not* meant to cure major illnesses or to treat serious health issues. In those circumstances, ideally a person should work in tandem with their allopathic doctor and a qualified BioSET practitioner. However, if applied correctly, these home treatments can help to alleviate sensitivities to many ordinary substances to which a person is sensitive, improving their digestion and over-all health and, hopefully, decreasing their asthma symptoms and their reliance on medications.

The samples or vials used in this procedure will represent the substances that are stressing the person and causing sensitivities and reactions. If their muscle goes weak when holding any of these samples, it may mean that their energy system is reacting negatively to the presence of that substance.

In order to begin a BioSET home sensitivity clearing, you will need the following:

1. A subject who wishes to receive a sensitivity clearing. The subject can be a friend or family member or even yourself. Instructions for self-testing and for self-clearings are included elsewhere in this chapter.

2. A quiet room shut away from any activities that might distract from your clearing, such as ringing phones or children.

3. A sample (or vial) of the item(s) that need to be tested and cleared.

For best results, clear the person for one item at a time. Often, it is tempting to combine items to speed up the process, but my experience has taught me that the body responds much more completely to substances when they are cleared one at a time.

This home clearing can be used to clear sensitivities to foods, collected pollen, dust, fabrics, swimming pool water, cosmetics, toothpaste, and many other substances (see chapter 11 for more details).

STEP 1: PREPARING THE ORDER OF TESTING

At this point it is necessary to determine the order in which the sensitivities will be cleared. Although BioSET home clearings are an ideal way to clear individual substances, it is more effective to clear sensitivities according to the order described in this chapter. Clearing the basic ten sensitivities first will take care of the majority of common problem foods. The ten basic sensitivities are

+ Amino acids
+ Phenolics
+ Biochemicals
+ Minerals
+ Vitamin C
+ B vitamins
+ Sugars
+ Vitamin A
+ Vitamin E
+ Fatty acids

If you don't have a sample kit of these items, just begin with the items to which the person suspects they are sensitive. You can make your own sample vials using empty sterile glass vials. They should be composed of thin glass (the glass in a spice bottle, for example, is too thick). A wineglass or small glass cup can also be used to contain an item—the thinner the glass, the better. (See appendix B for information on purchasing empty glass vials.)

You can also order samples of especially prepared items, produced according to the standards of the Federal Homeopathic Pharmacopoeia of the United States. These vials are excellent for use in BioSET sensitivity clearings. (Information on ordering a kit of vials can be found through www.bioset.com.)

STEP 2: PREPARING THE SUBJECT

Have the subject drink a glass of water to balance their energy. This ensures that your test results will be more reliable.

It is almost impossible to muscle test children under five years of age, but the clearings work wonderfully on them, so just skip Step 1 and then follow steps 2 through 4 to clear the child for suspected sensitivities. As I mentioned before, there's no harm in clearing someone for something to which they are not actually sensitive. Since the BioSET clearings consist of gentle acupressure massage, the massage tends to be relaxing and restorative even if you do not select the correct sensitivity.

STEP 3: TESTING THE SUBJECT

Place an item sample in the subject's hand, and do a muscle test, following the instructions given earlier in this chapter. If the subject tests strong with the sample in their hand, that substance is not a stressor and you can move on to the next substance. If the item tests weak, a BioSET sensitivity clearing is needed. If you are using a BioSET kit, you can clear items according to the sequence in the kit.

The clearing procedure is the same for all substances that test as sensitivities. Remember, in all cases, a strong response means that no clearings are necessary and a weak response means that the substance causes physical stress and needs a clearing.

STEP 4: USING THE ACUPRESSURE TECHNIQUE FOR BIOSET CLEARING

When a testing shows a weak muscle response, indicating a sensitivity that should be cleared, the vial or sample containing the substance should remain in the patient's hand. For example, if muscle testing points to a sensitivity to chocolate, the patient should continue to hold the chocolate during clearing.

The BioSET clearing for sensitivities has two parts:

+ Part I: Acupressure gently applied to the back
+ Part II: Gentle pressure on a series of nineteen acupressure points on the arms and legs

PART I: PERFORMING ACUPRESSURE ON THE BACK

You can learn to perform gentle acupressure on a person's back quickly and effectively, even without previous training in bodywork. Begin by locating the acupressure points on the patient's back; they are about an inch on either side of the vertebrae, the spinal ridges that run from the top of the neck to the base of the spine. You will be working on twenty-three pairs of points. During the clearing, the patient must continue to hold the vial containing the sensitive substance.

You can perform the BioSET Acupressure Technique using your fingertips, knuckles, or thumbs, whichever works best for you. For convenience, I will use the word "thumbs" in the following description.

Applying light pressure, rotate your thumbs in a clockwise motion about three times to stimulate each point. My experience suggests that three repetitions on each point will be enough for most people, although there is no fixed

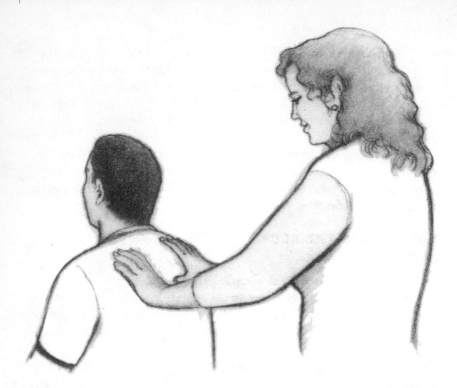

number of times necessary for appropriate stimulation. Since the changes you are trying to effect require very little stimulation, you can ease your pressure if the acupressure creates any discomfort for your subject.

Massage all of twenty-three sets of points in the clearing sequence in the same way. You can save time by using both thumbs to stimulate both sides of the spine simultaneously. Perform the gentle acupressure series four times, as the patient uses each one of the following four breathing techniques: holding the breath, exhaling, panting, and breathing normally.

Stage 1: *Holding the breath.* The subject should take a deep breath and hold it in while you move down the spine, stimulating the acupressure points on either side of the spinal column. Pause whenever your subject needs to take another breath. Resume acupressure as soon as the subject begins to hold their breath again.

Stage 2: *Exhaling.* The second time you stimulate all the acupressure points, the subject should exhale slowly and gradually.

Stage 3: *Panting breath.* The third time you stimulate the acupressure points, the subject should pant as quickly and vigorously as she can. Although asthmatics and people with respiratory problems may have difficulty sustaining this kind of breathing, the clearing can still be effective, even if the breathing pattern is broken. They should proceed carefully, panting only as long as they remain comfortable.

Stage 4: *Breathing normally.* On the fourth repetition, your subject should breathe normally as you stimulate the series of acupressure points along the spinal column.

Following the acupressure, retest your subject for a muscle response, making sure that the subject is still holding the sample. The muscle will resist your pressure if the clearing has succeeded, indicating that sensitivity to the substance has probably been cleared. Repeat the clearing if the subject's muscle test remains weak.

After retesting, you may find that you need to repeat a clearing once or twice; it is not unusual for a subject to require some repetition, although the first clearing is successful about 90 percent of the time when testing and clearing have been performed correctly. Don't worry about the need to repeat a clearing; just repeat the acupressure technique until the muscle tests strong.

In some cases, a person cannot be desensitized by home treatments. Various factors may be influencing the effectiveness of the clearings. When a case is more complicated, you should consult a trained BioSET practitioner. You can locate a practitioner near you by checking the list posted on the BioSET website at www.bioset.net.

PART II: STIMULATING THE NINETEEN KEY ACUPRESSURE POINTS

To stimulate energy flow throughout the body, apply the BioSET Acupressure Technique described above to the nineteen standard acupressure points shown in the illustrations on the facing page. As you perform the acupressure, your subject can assist the clearing by continuing to hold a sample of the allergen in a vial, in order to clear any blockages in the body's electromagnetic energetic system.

Referring to the list of acupressure points and the diagrams that follow, begin this part of the procedure on the right side of the subject's body, starting with the acupressure point on the hand. Work through the points, moving in a clockwise direction, until you complete the circuit by returning to your starting point. You should end your acupressure treatment on the same point with which you began. With the exception of one point, GV 20, on top of the head, all the points are paired and have exactly the same location on both

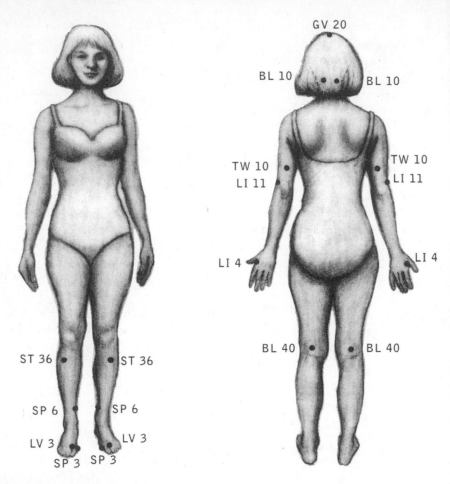

the right and left side of the body. I use the acupressure designations from traditional Chinese medicine to identify the points described below.

A Description of the Nineteen BioSET Acupressure Points

LI 4, right: Near the webbing between the thumb and index finger on the back of the right hand.

LI 11, right: In the depression between the right elbow and the end of the elbow crease.

TW 10, right: In the depression just above the right elbow on the back of the right arm.

BL 10, right: At the back of the head, about one inch to the right of the spine, in the center of the large muscle just below the bony ridge at the base of the skull.

GV 20: If you can imagine a line that runs from the tip of one ear over the head to the tip of the other ear, this point is on top of the head, exactly at the midpoint of the line.

BL 10, left: At the back of the head, about one inch to the left of the spine, in the center of the large muscle just below the bony ridge at the base of the skull.

TW 10, left: In the depression just above the left elbow on the back of the left arm.

LI 11, left: In the depression between the left elbow and the end of the elbow crease.

LI 4, left: Near the webbing between the thumb and index finger on the back of the left hand.

BL 40, left: In the middle of the large crease directly behind the left knee.

ST 36, left: About two to three inches (three or four finger widths) directly below the lower edge of the left kneecap and directly in line with the little toe.

SP 6, left: On the inside of the left leg, about two inches above the anklebone, in the soft tissue just behind the tibia (the larger of the two bones in the lower leg).

LIV 3, left: In the depression between the first and second tarsal bones (the big toe and second toe) of the left foot.

SP3, left: In the arch of the left foot, closest to the big toe.

SP3, right: In the arch of the right foot, closest to the big toe.

LIV 3, right: In the depression between the first and second tarsal bones (the big toe and second toe) of the right foot.

SP 6, right: On the inside of the right leg, about two inches above the anklebone, in the soft tissue just behind the tibia (the larger of the two bones in the lower leg).

ST 36, right: About two to three inches (three or four finger widths) directly below the lower edge of the right kneecap and directly in line with the little toe.

BL 40, right: In the middle of the large crease directly behind the right knee.

It should take you about fifteen minutes to complete the entire circuit. As you perform the acupressure, your subject can use the time for meditation and balance. Don't be concerned if they happen to fall asleep during the procedure.

When you have completed the circuit, your subject should remain comfortably relaxed for fifteen minutes, still holding the sample in their hand.

To perform self-clearings, you only need to follow Part II, applying acupressure on yourself for the nineteen points.

Stage 1: *Testing.* Use the O-ring method described earlier in this chapter to test yourself, making sure that your sample or vial comes in contact with your body. You can repeat this procedure to identify various sensitivities that need to be cleared.

Stage 2: *Applying acupressure to the nineteen points.* Omit Part I of the clearing since you cannot stimulate the back points on your own back by yourself. Perform Part II, completing the series six times, once every fifteen minutes over the course of approximately one and a half hours. You must continue to hold each sample in one hand for the entire series, using the fingers of that hand as needed for working on that side of the body. You can perform the self-clearings while you are reading or watching TV or a movie, but try to refrain from activities that would make it difficult to hold the samples for the entire time.

Stage 3: *Retesting.* Retest yourself at the end of the clearing cycle, keeping the vial or sample in your hand. You should now test strong in response to the item.

It may take several complete clearings to eliminate sensitivities to certain foods, cat hair, or pollen that have been bothering you for some time. One former patient of mine, Susan, who is a dedicated self-clearer, reports that her milk sensitivity was so great that it took her eleven self-clearings, one a day, to finally clear herself. Fortunately, she is now fully desensitized, and she can eat all dairy products without reacting to them. If you have persistent difficulty clearing a sensitivity, you should consult a BioSET practitioner.

Saliva Clearing

When immediate clearing is desired—at the first signs of symptoms, such as a runny nose, cough, or slight fever—an individual can be cleared for their own saliva. The symptomatic person, while holding a glass vial or jar containing their saliva, should have another person perform acupressure alongside their spine. This is followed by acupressure on the points indicated in the diagram (see p. 153) beginning with the right hand and progressing around the body clockwise three times and ending with the right hand. Light pressure is applied in a circular motion, with at least eight circles applied at each point.

Performed at the immediate onset of symptoms and every two to three hours thereafter if necessary, this clearing hastens the body's response to fight a virus or bacteria and generally leads to an elimination of symptoms within six to eight hours or often sooner.

BioSET Clearings: Different Protocols for Different Types of Asthma

After the ten basic sensitivities have been cleared, a BioSET practitioner can choose to follow a protocol of clearings based on the type of asthma a patient has. Seven basic types of asthma are described in this chapter:

+ Mild intermittent asthma
+ Mild persistent asthma
+ Moderate or severe persistent asthma
+ Occupational environment sensitivities (asthma-related)
+ Exercise-related asthma
+ Childhood asthma
+ Asthma in infants

In the sections that follow I discuss the different types of asthma and the characteristic BioSET protocols for clearings.

Mild Intermittent Asthma

Mild intermittent asthmatics are those with mild and infrequent symptoms. They may have attacks two or three times a year, usually triggered by viruses. Their symptoms tend to occur in spring and fall, when pollens proliferate. After clearing the basic sensitivities for people with mild asthma, practitioners begin working on the food sensitivities that did not clear automatically when the basics were cleared.

FOODS

Significant food sensitivities often seen in mild, intermittent asthmatics include cow's milk, fish, various nuts, seeds, soy and soy products, wheat, and citrus fruits. Other sensitivities to watch out for are chocolate, coffee, caffeine, many grains, spices, animal and vegetable fat, dried beans, yeast products, alcohol, baking powder, baking soda, gum mix, vegetable mix, and acidic and alkaline foods. Common acidic foods are sugars, starches, milk products, dairy products, fruits, vegetables, beans, tomatoes, onions, peppers, and potatoes, which are in the nightshade family. Often practitioners will clear for solanine, a chemical that is found in nightshade vegetables—tomatoes, capsicum, eggplant, tobacco, and potatoes. All of the nightshades contain nicotine, so practitioners sometimes will clear for it as well.

Clearing for mold can sometimes clear sensitivities to foods such as dried fruit, nuts, and cream cheese, and clearing for gluten can clear sensitivities to the grains that contain it—wheat, rye, oats, malt, and barley.

Corn is another common food sensitivity to check at this point in the clearing. Some commercial adhesives, talcum powder, and starched clothes can all provoke reactions in corn-sensitive patients. Sweat causes some of the corn-laden starch in clothing to be absorbed into the body and may provoke a reaction in asthmatics. Even licking a stamp can cause a reaction in an asthmatic who is sensitive to corn. Clearing a sensitivity to corn may clear sensitivities to many environmental sensitivities as well.

When clearing at home for a food, you can use the food itself in a thin glass such as a wineglass or a vial. Or, if you purchase a food kit, it may include the food item. (See appendix B for more detail.)

INGESTANTS: DOPAMINE AND SULFITES

When clearing a mild, intermittent asthmatic, practitioners will next look at a chemical neurotransmitter called dopamine, which stimulates the chemical neurotransmitter norepinephrine and is found in oranges and grapefruits. It causes problems in some asthmatics, as do salicylates and sulfites, which are found in many foods.

Sulfites prevent the browning and discoloration of foods that usually occurs at room temperature, and they are used to preserve wine, raw potatoes, and fresh vegetables. Ingesting large amounts of these chemicals can cause problems. By clearing or desensitizing people to sulfites, many other foods may clear, for example, avocados, baked products, beet sugar, dried fruits, fresh shrimp, fruit drinks, gelatin, wine, beer, potatoes, starches, vegetables, salads, and cider—even a sensitivity to cellophane. Sulfites are commonly used in the manufacture of many drugs, including asthma aerosols.

FOOD ADDITIVES

Food additives should be checked next. BHA, BHT, sodium benzoine, sodium nitrate, sodium sulfate, tartrazine, and food dyes are common problems. By clearing them, BioSET practitioners can clear sensitivities to foods that contain these additives.

INGESTANTS: OXALIC ACID

Clearing for oxalic acid can clear foods high in oxylates, including chocolate, caffeine, coffee, tomatoes, citrus fruits, spinach, some beans, and mushrooms. (See appendix A for a more complete list.)

If you are doing at-home self-clearings, vials containing sulfites, food additives, oxalic acid, and neurotransmitters may be difficult to find on your own. Check appendix B for help in locating these vials.

ENVIRONMENTAL SENSITIVITIES

After they have been cleared for foods, most mild, intermittent asthmatics are significantly improved and may feel they require less medication (this is something that needs to be discussed with and approved by your physician). In many cases, most of the foods clear when the ten basic sensitivities (amino acids, biochemicals, fatty acids, minerals, phenolics, sugars, vitamin A, B vitamins, vitamin C, and vitamin E) are cleared; therefore, each food does not have to be cleared individually. However, some more severe mild asthmatics need to be cleared for sensitivities to pollens, trees, dust, grasses, weeds, and shrubs, as well as for sensitivities to fabrics, including cotton and some nylons. Smoke, tobacco smoke, perfumes, animal dander, and molds may also need to be cleared.

When you are clearing at home for pollens, I recommend leaving a bowl of water outside your house. In fact, put bowls at different areas outside your house. After forty-eight hours, bring in the water with the pollen it has accumulated. (This technique can also be used indoors to collect mold, chemicals, and so on.) Then test yourself with this water to see if it causes a weak muscle response. If so, do a BioSET home self-clearing. Doing this every two weeks during high pollen season may be very helpful for those with hay fever symptoms, sinus congestion, and asthma.

If you need to clear a sensitivity to a fabric, holding the fabric while clearing is perfectly acceptable. As far as dust, which you usually can't see, vacuum the house, *especially* under your mattress, immediately before clearing and then test for a response. If there is one, then do a clearing on the dust. Put it into a vial, glass, or baby food jar to hold while clearing.

TWO PATIENT STORIES

One woman with mild intermittent asthma who came to see me suffered from asthma whenever she was around animals, tobacco smoke, and certain foods. As long as she stayed away from those items to which she was sensitive, she was generally free from episodes without taking medications. She was afraid of sudden attacks, however, and carried an inhaler while traveling in case of emergency. After we had cleared her for the basic sensitivities, she no longer needed an inhaler around animals or smoke. She has now been clear for many years, and she feels secure enough to travel without an inhaler.

One fourth-grade boy came to me with severe environmental sensitivities to pollen and trees and with mild asthma around cats. Mold, however, seemed to be his worst sensitivity, causing wheezing, congestion, hyperactivity, attention deficit disorder, and fatigue. We cleared him for the ten basic sensitivities and then for some foods—wheat, yeast, milk, and some fruits. After that, he was fine during the spring and summer high-pollen seasons and had no more reaction to cats. The dark circles under his eyes lightened quite a bit, and his attention span improved 100 percent, which was reflected in his grades.

Mild Persistent Asthma

Mild persistent asthmatics develop symptoms more frequently than mild intermittent asthmatics. They tend to experience problems every four to six weeks and use asthma medication every day in order to prevent symptoms.

PHENOLICS AND CHEMICALS PRODUCED BY THE IMMUNE SYSTEM

BioSET practitioners will start by clearing these types of asthma sufferers for the ten basic sensitivities and follow with a clearing for phenolics. They will also include clearings for histamine and prostaglandins, which are chemicals involved in the body's immune response to sensitivities. When a sensitivity or nonspecific irritant contacts the particular type of immune cells known as mast cells, the mast cells begin to leak histamine and prostaglandins into the surrounding tissue. These chemicals can cause muscle contractions, swelling, and mucus secretion. A sensitivity to these chemicals can have serious repercussions for an asthmatic.

INFECTANTS

Next practitioners will clear mild persistent asthmatics for sensitivities to infectants, including viruses, bacteria, fungi, and parasites. By clearing for the various infectants, we can prevent the cycle of chronic infections and chronic antibiotic use. With these infections out of the way, the lung tissue can have a chance to heal and the immune system can have a chance to strengthen.

CANDIDA

Yeast and fungi such as candida, in all its many forms, are a chronic sensitivity in both mild persistent and moderate or severe persistent asthmatics. Most asthmatics suffer the symptoms of candida—bloating, fatigue, and occasional vaginal infections. Yeast organisms have the ability to convert sugars to a chemical called pyruvate, which is then converted to acetaldehyde and carbon dioxide. Carbon dioxide is the main culprit in bloating and gas and can also be a problem for asthmatics.

When a patient is cleared for yeast or fungi, they also should be cleared for alcohol. Some scientific studies have shown that *Candida albicans* in the body can produce enough ethanol to make the infected individual drunk. Ethanol, which is in the phenolics group, can sometimes be cleared by clearing for phenolics.

When a patient has been cleared for the ten basic sensitivities, including phenolics, and some infectants, particularly candida, many respiratory problems decrease significantly and mild persistent asthmatics may require less medication.

When people are cleared for a sensitivity to candida, they should remain on a special diet for ten to fourteen days and curtail their sexual activity (or use a latex barrier) to ensure that candida is not passed back and forth sexually. Candida can also be spread through toothbrushes, dentures, fabrics, and skin-to-skin contact. If a couple goes to see a BioSET practitioner, the one displaying symptoms is usually the one who is sensitive. The person not demonstrating symptoms could still be passing candida to his or her mate, so both should be checked and, if needed, cleared. This is not absolutely essential, though, because once the candida sensitivity is successfully cleared, the symptoms of sensitivity to that yeast should not reoccur, even if candida is transmitted by another.

It takes as long as two months to completely balance a system that has been affected by candida, but the ten- to fourteen-day diet is crucial. The pathogenicity, or the infectant's ability to do harm, is a result of a sensitivity to that infectant. If people are not sensitive to candida, their bodies will be able to deal with it and eliminate it from the system.

Candida albicans and *Candidus tropicales* are the most common yeast infectants found in asthmatics. *Candida albicans* will grow rapidly in a medium of sugars, biotin, and organic salts, and prefers an acid pH. The higher the biotin level, the more the yeast. Antibiotics tend to increase the toxicity of yeast and candida. In fact, the widespread use of tetracycline antibiotic for teenage acne could end up causing more skin problems in the long run by encouraging yeast overgrowth.

Candida adheres to mucosal epithelial surfaces in the respiratory tract and provokes an antibody response in those who are sensitive. It has been shown to stimulate histamine release from mast cells, producing a strong sensitivity response that is a trigger for asthmatics.

Candida overgrowth occurs in the human body when immune defenses are locally impaired, such as a disturbance of the gut flora. This disturbance can be caused by parasitic, viral, or bacterial infections. Nutritional deficiencies, sensitivities, altered glucose metabolism, hypoglycemia, and diabetes can also be factors. Therapies such as antibiotics, cortical steroids, and oral contraceptives are factors in lowering immune defenses. Immunity may also be impaired by HIV infections, chemotherapy, radiation, genetic defects, high chemical exposure, high carbohydrate and sugar diets, pregnancy, menses, and thyroid and adrenal deficiencies.

Other symptoms of candida sensitivity in asthmatics are fatigue, moodiness, depression, anxiety, inability to concentrate, lack of energy, increased PMS symptoms in women, aching muscles and joints, arthritis, fibromyalgia, abdominal bloating, constipation, diarrhea and irritable bowel, skin rashes, vaginal and rectal itching, urticaria, cystitis, and persistent vaginal discharge. A significant number of asthmatics also have other ear, nose, and throat symptoms, recurrent ear infections, throat mucus, postnasal drip, and sinusitis. In males a correlation has been shown between chronic candida and prostatitis. Both male and female candida sufferers experience an unusual degree of craving for sweets and carbohydrates.

To clear a sensitivity to candida, it is necessary to have effectively cleared sensitivities to sugars and B vitamins. Following a clearing, patients follow a sugar- and carbohydrate-free diet that includes meat, vegetables, and unsweetened yogurt.

When undergoing treatments for candida, including antifungal medication or dietary changes, many people have what is called a die-off reaction, which means they may feel worse for a time before they get better. BioSET practitioners have found that this can be prevented by doing clearings for candida.

One man in his forties came to the BioSET clinic with chronic candida infections. He experienced fatigue, insomnia, severe bloating, and fogginess. He had suffered for a long time and tried many therapies, with only occasional and temporary relief. The woman he was with was also plagued with candida, so they were passing the problem back and forth. We cleared him for the ten basic sensitivities and then for candida and some other fungi to which he was sensitive. It took several sessions to clear his sensitivity. Then he went on the special diet for ten to fourteen days, and began taking a probiotic and a carbohydrate digestive that I prescribed. After clearings that stretched over a six-week period of time, he felt better.

Not every mild persistent asthmatic is sensitive to candida; however, certain conditions and symptoms put people at risk for this infection. People who have taken large amounts of antibiotics are at risk. People with chronic ear infections, athlete's foot, nail infections, skin rashes, oral thrush, colic, recurrent cystitis, jock itch, or loss of libido are likely to have candida infections, as are people who suffer from sensitivities during infancy and childhood, diabetes, or AIDS. If a person's symptoms start to manifest after taking oral contraceptives, that is a good indication of a possible candida sensitivity. Vaginal thrush, pelvic inflammatory disease (PID), and endometriosis can all indicate candida. Recurring nasal polyps may also indicate a candida and/or a mold sensitivity. Fortunately, all of these conditions can be cleared effectively with BioSET.

Immunosuppressive drugs such as steroids, cortisone, and prednisone for asthma, skin problems, or arthritis can all contribute to a candida sensitivity. Mild persistent and moderate or severe persistent asthmatics are likely to have taken these medications at one time or another. Another sign of sensitivity is when one's symptoms are aggravated after eating foods containing yeast or molds, or if the symptoms get worse during wet weather, on humid days, or after exposure to dampness in places such as cellars and attics. Candida infections may cause a craving for sweets, alcohol, and carbohydrates, but this may also be caused by sensitivities to sugars or B vitamins. High sugar diets and multiple pregnancies can bring on a candida sensitivity.

VIRUSES, BACTERIA, AND PARASITES

Other groups of infectants for which BioSET practitioners clear are parasites, bacteria, and viruses, which can cause symptoms ranging from asthma to fatigue.[1] (See chapter 5 for further information on infectants.) Some of the infectants BioSET practitioners routinely check for are giardia, camplobactor, entero viruses, and Heliobactor pylori, the last of which is related to ulcers and can be a problem for elderly asthmatics. Asthmatics as a group tend to respond well to clearings for parasites and bacteria. Bacterial clearings may turn the corner for a mild persistent asthmatic. Practitioners have found from fifteen to twenty bacterial sensitivities in mild persistent asthmatics.

Home treatment of infectants is not recommended unless a person is performing a saliva clearing for acute viruses, colds, or flu. The only exception is if you are *already* under a BioSET practitioner's supervision, in which case, home clearings can hasten the course of your clearings.

FOODS

When a patient has been cleared for parasites, BioSET practitioners will then move on to food sensitivities. Practitioners will do detailed and ongoing testing on each patient to find and clear all of their food sensitivities.

ENVIRONMENTAL SENSITIVITIES

From foods, BioSET practitioners then begin to test for environmental sensitivities, such as pollens, molds, and other outdoor elements; animal dander; dust; fabrics; wood; chemical irritants; gas in the house; or other indoor irritants. Any of these can be triggers for asthmatics.

In a process called "outgassing," certain products give off gases or chemicals that can be absorbed into the bloodstream through touch or inhalation. Things such as perfume, new carpets, heated plastic, and even flowers on a table all outgas. Many of these gases can be smelled, but chemicals without smell can also be toxic or deadly triggers for asthmatics. Materials in car interiors, formaldehyde, toluene, zylene, hexanes, perochloroethylene, nitrous oxide, ozone, carbon monoxide, carbon dioxide, alkanes, petrochemicals, and other hydrocarbons can all be health threats to asthmatics and other sensitive people. Photocopy paper can outgas trichloroethylene (TCE), which is also a solvent used in dry cleaning fluids, carpet shampoos, floor polishes, and furniture glues. Asthmatics should be desensitized to this chemical in particular. Paint fumes may be a problem, along with cleaning solvents, aerosol sprays, and tobacco and wood smoke.

If a patient is not completely sure which chemical in a room is causing a problem, BioSET practitioners will advise the individual to put out a small jar of water and leave it open for forty-eight hours. Then the person should close the jar, bring it in to the clinic, and let the practitioner clear them for a sensitivity to whatever outgassed chemicals are trapped in the water. Patients can follow the same procedure with suspected outdoor sensitivities by putting a bowl of water outside their house to collect pollen for forty-eight hours, bringing the water to the clinic, and having the practitioner clear them for whatever is in the water. Sometimes BioSET practitioners still need to clear for individual sensitivities, such as the specific molds and mildew in a patient's bathroom. However, when practitioners clear for an inhalant, such as tobacco smoke or perfume, they will have the patient inhale the substance, rather than just touch it during the session.

Environmental sensitivities are usually the last ones that need to be cleared for mild persistent asthmatics. Some individuals also need to be cleared for cortisol, adrenaline, or other hormones, including male or female hormones. At this point in the clearing, the mild persistent asthmatic should be free of symptoms.

Moderate or Severe Persistent Asthma

Moderate or severe persistent asthmatics are people who experience frequent acute asthmatic episodes. They wheeze and cough regularly, need daily clearings and medication, and find exercise and sports difficult.

INGESTANTS: MEDICATIONS

For moderate and severe asthmatics, BioSET practitioners begin by clearing the ten basic sensitivities. Practitioners next clear for infectants. Clearing for candida is crucial, along with clearing for parasites and bacteria. Sensitivities to bacteria are probably the most serious problems for severe asthmatics. These bacteria may produce massive amounts of mucus, establishing an environment for chronic infections, possibly leading to chronic bronchitis.

Much of the problem with bacterial overgrowth is often the direct result of years of antibiotic abuse[2] in combination with immunosuppressive drugs like prednisone and other corticosteroids. Clearing asthmatics for bacterial sensitivities often produces increased stamina and energy levels and a reduction of other sensitivities.

FOODS AND ENVIRONMENTAL SENSITIVITIES

Practitioners also check for sensitivities in every food and food group. Some food sensitivities may clear when the ten basic sensitivities have been cleared, but there are still many other foods to clear for. During pollen season BioSET practitioners clear for pollens.

FOOD ADDITIVES: PESTICIDES

Next BioSET practitioners clear for pesticides, which include insecticides, fungicides, herbicides, fumigants, and rodenticides. There are several families of insecticides: organophosphates, chlorinated hydrocarbons, botanicals, and chemical sterilants.

One asthmatic man who visited the BioSET clinic did extremely well after he had been cleared for all of the ten basic sensitivities and pollens. He had not needed to use medications for months, that is, until he visited his father, whose house had just been fumigated by a pest control firm. Because the pesticide residues were lingering in the house, he experienced a severe asthmatic attack and had to go to the hospital, where he was prescribed steroids. After he was cleared for the pesticides, he recovered almost immediately and no longer had any problems with his father's house.

Although DDT was banned as toxic many years ago, it still lingers in the soil and we continue to be exposed to it. Also, some of the so-called inert ingredients in commercial pesticides are among the most harmful. Carbon tetrachloride and chloroform, for example, are powerful liver and central nervous system toxins. Fruits are sprayed with a pesticide called daminozide, which is potentially harmful for asthmatics. Even natural repellents such as vinegar and garlic can be toxic to anyone who is allergic to them.

Authorities are reluctant to issue warnings about specific pesticide exposure levels, because exact toxic levels are not known. Measuring pesticide levels in one food would not be an accurate measure of a health hazard, anyway, since chemical combinations can have a synergistic effect. Pesticides can also leak into water supplies, so BioSET practitioners always check clients for sensitivity to the water they drink, whether it is spring water, filtered water, or tap water.

Just because people have been desensitized to pesticides, however, does not mean that these chemicals are no longer harmful. Ingesting them can still cause cancer, liver damage, stomach problems, or other symptoms. Washing fruits and vegetables is generally not an effective way to get rid of pesticides. Certain natural products, such as grapefruit extract and borax, can be used to remove pesticides, but people should make sure they are not sensitive to those products before using them. By far, the best way to avoid pesticides is to eat organically grown food.

INHALANTS: PERFUMES AND COSMETICS

After pesticides, BioSET practitioners next clear for perfumes and cosmetics, which can be a trigger for asthmatics. Some of the common ingredients that cause trouble are alcohol; aluminum; the acetone found in nail polish remover; ammonium compounds; chloride, a preservative used in some cosmetics to prevent the growth of bacteria; BHA, a synthetic antioxidant; mercury; and colorants, dyes, and color additives that contain coal tar substances. These chemicals can also be a cause of hyperactivity in children. Other potentially sensitive products are detergents, soaps, petroleum derivatives, fluorinated hydrocarbons used in aerosols, mineral oils, crude oil, and liquid hydrocarbon, found in hair sprays—a potential problem for both hairdressers and clients. In all, cosmetics and toiletries contain about eight thousand chemicals and chemical compounds, many of which have not been tested by the FDA.

For asthmatics, perfumes and cosmetics, which are derived from petroleum or coal tar, can be as bad as cigarette smoke. Even flower oils are chemically extracted with petroleum ether. Unfortunately, it is becoming impossible to walk into a store, wash clothes, or flush a toilet without being assailed by scents and chemicals. Perfumes can linger in the air, on clothing, and on furniture in buses, theaters, restaurants, and workplaces long after the person wearing them has gone. An effective air purifier (see appendix B for more information on water and air filters) can be helpful in reducing the exposure to tolerable levels.

Fragrances are among the few chemicals in products for human use that are not regulated, even though they pose an extreme danger to many people. There should be clear labeling with precise information about ingredients and restrictions on chemicals used in scented products.

CONTACTANTS

Next practitioners will clear moderate and severe persistent asthmatics for sensitivities to contactants.

FABRICS

The next group of sensitivities for which moderate or severe asthmatics are always tested is fabrics. This includes cotton, rayon, nylon, Dacron, polyester, and acrylic. Clearing for these fabrics is crucial for those asthmatics with severe sinus problems, difficulty smelling or tasting, sinus congestion, runny nose, wheezing, and frequent night attacks.

CHEMICALS IN HOUSEHOLD PRODUCTS

Next BioSET practitioners clear for chemicals found in household products, home and work spaces, public places, and cars. We clear for formaldehyde, which is synthesized from methyl alcohol and is found in insulation, particleboard, foam rubber, detergents, carpet underlay, new clothes and other textiles, newsprint, household and industrial cleaners, propellants, plywood, resin, glue, concrete, and dyes. It is also found in name tags, correction fluids, leather goods, decaffeinated coffee, and embalming fluid.

INHALANTS: CARBON DIOXIDE AND OZONE

After clearing a patient for chemicals, a practitioner next clears them for carbon dioxide and ozone. This is especially important for those asthmatics whose symptoms get worse when they climb to the top of a mountain or fly in airplanes, times when the body produces more carbon dioxide. Candida can also produce a lot of carbon dioxide, which creates bloating. For people who are sensitive to carbon dioxide, any excess can stress the immune system.

MISCELLANEOUS SENSITIVITIES

BioSET practitioners next clear for any miscellaneous sensitivities for which a patient has tested positive. These might include Freon from air-conditioning, radon, plants and ferns, various gums, kapok from mattresses, poison oak and poison ivy, rubber, adhesive tape, cement, chalk, all pesticides, hydrocarbons, paper mix, newsprint, photocopy paper, plastics, radiation, benzene, labels, nail chemicals, hair chemicals, and bug spray.

HORMONES

Practitioners will also check for sensitivities to hormones, such as adrenaline, estrogen, testosterone, progesterone, thyroid, and cortisol, the natural inflammatory that reacts to sensitivities in the body. People who are sensitive to cortisol may have an asthmatic attack in response to an inflammation caused by another sensitivity. Checking other adrenal hormones such as insulin, glucagon, and DHEA is also important. Women who become more asthmatic during PMS are usually sensitive to progesterone. If their symptoms increase during and immediately after the menstrual cycle, they are probably sensitive to estrogen. These sensitivities respond well to BioSET clearings.

Practitioners have found that many asthmatics who experience fatigue, temperature intolerance, weight gain, and depression, and test positive for candida sensitivity, are often deficient in thyroid hormones or sensitive to their own thyroid. A common name for this condition is autoimmune thyroiditis (Hashimoto's). This is the most common hypothyroid disorder. These individuals do well when cleared for the thyroid hormone, iodine, vegetable fat, animal fat, and some amino acids. This thyroid condition is common in people with moderate or severe persistent asthma, but it is more rare in those with mild intermittent asthma.

HISTAMINES: IMMUNE MEDIATORS

The next group of sensitivities for which practitioners test is the immune mediators. Mediators cause the walls of the bronchial tubes to swell up, and muscles may go into spasm, creating an obstruction in the lungs. There is the added danger that people may be sensitive to the mast cells and the mediators, one of which is histamine. There is also a newly discovered group called leukotrienes to which people can be sensitive.

When the mediators, histamine and prostaglandins, cause the smooth muscle to contract, the result is edema, swelling, and increased mucus secretion. This mucus production is intended as a defense against infectants, but it is also produced by sensitivity reactions when there are no infectants present. When this occurs, cells such as the eosinophils, lymphocytes, T cells, macrophages, epithelial cells, and neutrophils, which are in the bloodstream, move into the bronchial tube and attach themselves where the walls are inflamed. If the body is sensitive to any of those cells, a further reaction may occur to the bronchial tissue. The eosinophils play the biggest role in this reaction.

When the bronchial tube is totally inflamed, fibrin, a kind of scar tissue, is deposited in the bronchial tube to aid in healing, and the scarring causes the tubes to contract. A possible sensitivity to the fibrin will intensify the reaction. When these reactions occur, the bronchial tubes do not let air pass in and out of the lungs, resulting in the common symptoms of asthma. Therefore, clearing these sensitivities in asthmatics can be very helpful. Clearing sensitivities to mast cells and specific cell mediators, combined with extra doses of the anti-inflammatory enzyme protease, will be beneficial.

Many patients have found self-clearing at home to be effective at the onset of an asthma attack. Pressing the acupressure points (see the section on self-clearing in chapter 10) can soothe breathing, coughing, and wheezing and may prevent the development of a severe episode. But this procedure needs to be done *immediately*, even on the way to the physician or emergency room.

Recently, a woman patient who was an asthmatic developed a slight infection after a long airplane ride. Planes are a common place to pick up viruses because of the poor ventilation. I recommend that people do a saliva clearing right after getting off a plane to prevent sickness and distress. As soon as she arrived at her hotel, she did a self-clearing with her saliva and a virus vial, and also took some extra protease enzymes and vitamin C enzyme formula. She noticed a complete reversal of her symptoms within minutes. After following up with another saliva clearing before bed that night, her asthma was in complete control. This patient is indeed an advocate of self-clearing, and she believes that, in this case, it helped her to avoid a severe cough and asthma aggravation.

DIGESTIVE METABOLIC ENZYMES FOR ASTHMA

Sometimes it is also necessary to clear severe asthmatics with digestive and metabolic enzymes to support their metabolism, nutrient absorption, and the integrity of their immune system. These enzymes can have a profound effect on digestion and on building stamina and immune function. Digestion is key to any chronic health problem. Therefore, BioSET practitioners always test asthmatics before giving them enzymes to make sure they are not sensitive to them. If people are sensitive to enzymes, their digestion will usually be poor, and for asthmatics this can mean an accumulation of mucus from foods that trigger attacks. Taking enzyme supplements is not useful to people who are sensitive to them. So clearing for sensitivities to enzymes can be very critical in their therapy.

One patient with chronic stomach pain and heartburn had tried everything, without success. I found that she was sensitive to certain digestive enzymes. After clearing her for that sensitivity, she has not had a bout with heartburn in three months. She said, "You're a miracle worker. Nothing has ever worked for me before."

Occupational Environment Sensitivities

In all of the asthma groups—mild intermittent, mild persistent, and moderate or severe persistent—practitioners also clear for occupational environment sensitivities, substances people are frequently exposed to in the workplace. For example, if a person works in a gas station, we will clear for gas fumes, chemicals, gas, and diesel exhaust. If a patient is a painter, we will clear for paints, chemicals, and other work-related materials. We will clear a person who works in a hair salon for hair dyes, a photographer for photographic chemicals, people who work in detergent factories for chemicals that help remove stains, people who are artists for adhesives and epoxy resins, and bakers for dyes, flour, and cornstarch.

There are many other problem substances to which people are exposed in the workplace. Here is a list of the common ones:

+ Cannery workers are exposed to bleaches, chrome, fish parts, foods, and oils.

+ Carpenters are exposed to adhesives, exotic wood, plastics, fiberglass, and varnishes.

+ Chemists are exposed to antibiotics, formalines, acids, and ammonia.

+ Electricians are exposed to electricity and isocyanates.

+ Florists are exposed to mold.

+ Professional gardeners are exposed to dried pots, pollens, fertilizers, and mulch.

+ Garment workers are exposed to different fabrics: cotton, nylon, acrylic, polyester, feathers, formalines, and solvents.

+ Metal workers are exposed to platinum, chromates, and metal dusts.

+ Printers are exposed to cobalt, glue, solvents, zinc, chromates, gum arabic, and pine resin.

All of these are potential sensitivities and potential triggers for asthmatics. Many of these sensitivities can be cleared using either the actual substance or collecting water that has been exposed to it, as described earlier.

One client of mine worked in a bread store. He was an asthmatic and suffered from chronic sinus problems. When he was cleared of his wheat sensitivity, he no longer had problems being around bread. Clearing for occupational sensitivities such as those described above can keep people from having to leave work and go on disability.

Exercise-Induced Asthma

Exercise-induced asthma is a special kind of asthma that BioSET practitioners believe is caused by sensitivities to things people come into contact with while exercising. Some of these sensitivities include cold air, wind, hot air, humidity, and Freon. Carbon dioxide, oxygen, and adrenaline sensitivities can also bring on asthma, as can sensitivities to the body's own bronchial tubes, adrenals, sinus, or nasal mucosa. For athletes who wheeze when pollens are high, pollens may be one of the problems. Emotions related to stress can also be a problem for athletes. Other possibilities are mold and chemicals in pools, and dust in gymnasiums.

Food sensitivities may also play a big role in exercise-induced asthma. Home self-treatments can be of great assistance in this type of asthma. Athletes with this condition tend to have more rhinitis than other asthmatics and may not be able to smell or taste. They need to have clearings for sensitivities particular to the sinus cavity. Practitioners may also clear them for foods, environmental sensitivities, dust, and mold.

Asthma in Children and Infants

BioSET practitioners always test for the ten basic sensitivities with children diagnosed with asthma, then immediately test for food sensitivities unless the patient has chronic sinusitis, ear infections, or bronchitis, even though bronchitis is not as common in children as it is in adults. If the child has chronic ear infections, the practitioner will clear for infectants such as bacteria, viruses, and parasites. We have had extraordinary success clearing ear infections with BioSET. Extra protease is helpful in this case, and a child can easily ingest the protease with applesauce. The foods most likely implicated in ear infections are sugar, ice cream, and other dairy products. Soy and eggs can also be a problem.

BioSET practitioners also clear children for food additives such as sulfites and food coloring. Occasionally, a practitioner will also clear for pollens, trees, and grasses. However, children tend to have more severe sensitivities to foods than to the environment, which shows up again and again in tests and case histories. It usually takes less time for them than for adults to clear these sensitivities, and they are often medication-free after the first few clearings, especially after a clearing for vitamin C.

When infants are diagnosed with asthma, a BioSET practitioner will clear them for mother's milk or formula first. Sometimes these sensitivities clear up right away. Then the practitioner will begin clearing for the ten basic sensitivities and food. They will also check for vitamin C, sugar, and mold. We have found that alternaria, a common mold during the damp season, can be a severe sensitivity for children and infants.

Nocturnal Asthma

When asthma symptoms occur at night or in the early morning, the condition is called nocturnal asthma. Studies have repeatedly found that 90 percent of asthmatics wake up coughing and wheezing sometime during the night, most commonly between 3:00 and 5:00 a.m. According to acupuncture, this is the time when the lung meridian is most active.

A major consequence of nocturnal asthma is a loss of sleep, which can result in a deterioration of daytime performance and other symptoms associated with lack of sleep, such as attention deficit and problems with homework for children and work for adults. These problems affect other family members as well.

There are many possible explanations for nighttime asthma, and I have had many sleepless nights myself wondering about the possibilities. One possible explanation I have developed is that cortisone and epinephrine levels may fall during the period when an asthmatic awakens with symptoms. Cortisone combats inflammation while epinephrine causes bronchial constriction. Low levels may cause increased inflammation and bronchial inactivity, triggering an aggravation of symptoms. Another possible explanation is that gastric reflux—the regurgitation of food or acid from the stomach—is common at that time, especially in elderly people.

A third explanation is that while sleeping, people are exposed to common sensitivities that can trigger an asthma attack, such as fabrics, feathers, dust, and animal dander. A fourth possible explanation is related to the body's position while sleeping. Studies have shown that airway inflammation is more severe when people are lying down than when they are standing up.

Any of these factors could cause coughing or wheezing serious enough to wake up someone. Because the lung's bioenergetic pathway is most active at that time of the night, the organ may be more easily stimulated to react.

Conquering Asthma: The Healing Journey

The amount of time it takes to see improvement will vary for each person with asthma. Every individual is different, and every individual's program will be different too. In evaluating the program and making recommendations for different people, a practitioner needs to become familiar with their symptoms, history, immune response, and particular sensitivities. Everyone's response to BioSET is influenced by these factors.

People who identify themselves as moderate or severe persistent asthmatics may actually respond quickly, while those who think they are mild persistent may require extra clearings. BioSET practitioners are taught to treat the individual, not the disease, so the basic sequence is followed strictly and then modified based on an individual's sensitivities.

The healing may take time. For some asthmatics it takes a couple of months; for others it could take as long as two years. Consistency with home clearings, enzyme use, and a healthy lifestyle will expedite the healing and enable a reduction in suffering and medication. Asthmatics and people with other chronic disorders who pursue this approach will eventually find themselves feeling vastly improved. For example, a fourth-grade boy, John, came to the BioSET clinic with hay fever, multiple sensitivities, asthma, and about twenty warts on each hand and arm. We went through all ten basic clearings, then tackled foods, pollens, and environmental sensitivities. He then asked me if I could make his warts go away before the school year started. I told him practitioners had experienced very good results with warts and we could clear the virus that caused them with BioSET. I cleared John for the wart virus a couple of times, and then his mother did clearings on him at home. We did not see him for some time after that, due to the summer holiday break. But when school began again, he came to the clinic for a reevaluation. He walked into the office, and there was not one wart on his body. His skin was as smooth as silk, and the dark circles were gone from under his eyes as well. A couple of weeks after we had ended the clearing at the clinic, he told me, he woke up in the morning and found that he could start brushing off the warts. Within one week all his warts were gone. He had no more problems with mold or pollen, and he had been around cats and other animals without any reaction.

The lists of sensitivities discussed in this chapter and others are just examples. Asthmatics need to be tested and evaluated to find out exactly what their sensitivities are. This is done by observing their specific responses, testing suspect substances, and research, such as reading and rereading this book for other possible clues and tips for healing.

Stamina

Fatigue is often the result of sensitivities, poor digestion, and a collection of toxins that slow down the body. Most people react to low energy levels by drinking coffee, eating sugar, smoking cigarettes, or relying on other stimulants that give them a boost of energy. These short-term solutions may actually aggravate the problem, causing more complications and worsening chronic health problems. The maintenance of high levels of energy is achieved by

- Eliminating sensitivities
- Improving digestion and the absorption of nutrients
- Removing toxins from the body
- Increasing nutrients

Good energy levels, stamina, and a resistance to aging are all by-products of optimum health and homeostasis (a state of equilibrium).

Energy Level Indicators

Many things can hinder the maintenance of healthy energy levels. To determine the cause of low energy, BioSET practitioners do a health assessment with a detailed questionnaire, energetic muscle testing, or EAV (electro acupuncture) testing. These tools reveal many factors relating to energy levels. For information on a complete assessment, see *MicroMiracles: Discover the Healing Power of Enzymes.*

DIGESTION

The first indicator of a person's overall energy levels is the efficiency of their digestion and ability to absorb nutrients into the body. People can eat the healthiest of foods, but if they do not digest or absorb them properly, they cannot benefit from them because they are not utilizing the vitamins and minerals necessary for the body's metabolic functions and a healthy immune system.

Good digestion is the key to high energy levels, and problems with digestion differ from individual to individual. For example, some people are carbohydrate intolerant, and some are protein and fat intolerant.

When undigested food seeps into the bloodstream, it sets off an immune inflammatory reaction that, in turn, can cause an autoimmune or auto-aggressive response.[1] The undigested food also consumes essential metabolic enzymes needed to complete the process of digestion. The extra energy used in this process reduces the amount of energy gained from the foods. This is a principal cause of fatigue.

IMPAIRED THYROID FUNCTION

The next indicator of low energy is impaired thyroid function. This condition can result in a decrease in energy because the thyroid influences many other metabolic processes, hormonal processes, and tissue functioning in the body. Impaired adrenal function can have similar effects.

DEFICIENCIES AND SENSITIVITIES

Other possible causes of low energy levels include

+ Vitamin and mineral deficiencies resulting from poor absorption
+ Food sensitivities
+ Poor liver function
+ An overgrowth of yeast, bacteria, or parasites in the gastrointestinal system
+ Lack of sleep
+ Insufficient exercise
+ Mental and emotional illnesses and imbalances

Fatigue can also be caused by other medical problems and serious pathologies, so all possibilities of disease or physical dysfunction should be carefully evaluated.

In dealing with food and environmental sensitivities, it is helpful and appropriate to remove the food sensitivities from the diet and the environmental toxins from the person's surroundings. Because some sensitivities are extremely difficult to avoid, however, clearing with BioSET is an important alternative to permanent avoidance. Often food sensitivities can be eliminated by taking a digestive enzyme before meals.

Over time, hypersensitive reactions can inhibit good immune system function and impair energy levels and stamina. When a sensitivity is eradicated, the process of toxicity and immune system damage ends. Feeling tired after eating a particular food is a common experience that signals a sensitivity to that food. When a food sensitivity is cleared with either enzymes and/or BioSET clearings, a person will feel a change of energy either immediately or within fourteen days.

Yeast, bacteria, fungi, and parasite sensitivities in the intestinal system and bloodstream can overload the immune system and prevent it from protecting us from other nasty pathogens. Fatigue is a symptom of sensitivity to these substances. Sugar, carbohydrates in general, and alcohol all intensify the severity of these sensitivities. Taking a good probiotic (see chapter 13, Enzyme Therapy) and dietary changes with enzymes and BioSET clearings are essential solutions to these nagging predators.

TOXINS

Toxic buildup in the body is another common cause of fatigue. Toxins come from chemicals in our environment, food and environmental sensitivities, and by-products of the body's everyday metabolism. Smog and pesticides, food additives, alcohol, drinking water, medications, and drugs also can poison our systems. Sometimes these toxic buildups occur because the organs of elimination—skin, colon, lungs, and kidneys—are not working properly. Detoxification requires healthy digestion and elimination and an awareness of what we are putting into our bodies.

BioSET can be extremely helpful to the detoxification process. Effective detoxification can be achieved through a combination of desensitization to environmental sensitivities; reducing consumption of foods grown with pesticides, fungicides, and herbicides; and eliminating rancid fats, trans fats, carbohydrates, particularly grains,[2] and chemically prepared fats and margarine. Trans fats, margarine, and rancid oils contain partially hydrogenated oils that can interfere with the production of adenosine triphosphate (ATP), a substance in cellular metabolism that helps produce energy at the cellular level. Partially hydrogenated oils can also toxify the liver. Smoking and exposure to secondhand smoke should be avoided, and water should be filtered to remove chemicals such as chlorine, fluorine, and other toxins. Also, stimulants such as caffeine and sugars that lower energy, deplete vitamins and minerals such as potassium, and weaken the immune system should be avoided.

Improving Energy Levels

There are various ways to improve energy levels. Some of the most important are cleansing the liver and getting plenty of exercise. Interestingly, good posture and body alignment is also necessary for healthy energy.

LIVER DETOXIFICATION

The liver is an important organ in maintaining good energy levels and detoxifying the body. Good digestion, desensitization, and good nutrition keep the liver working optimally. In addition, the liver should be cleansed at least once or twice a year. (See appendix B for detoxification resources.)

A liver detoxification program works particularly well after a person has been cleared for the ten basic sensitivities (amino acids, biochemicals, fatty acids, minerals, phenolics, sugars, vitamin A, B vitamins, vitamin C, and vitamin E). When those sensitivities have been cleared, the person experiences fewer side effects or detoxification symptoms—such as headache, achiness, tiredness, skin rashes, irritability, and dizziness—and the cleansing is quicker and more effective. Liver cleansing is highly recommended for anyone with energy and stamina problems and for people with chronic health problems. I recommend doing it once or twice a year. It is also a great way to lose weight.

EXERCISE

Exercise is one of the most important factors in increasing energy levels because it transports more oxygen into the body through increased circulation. Higher oxygen levels help burn off sugars and fats in the body, which, in turn, can increase energy levels. Exercise also increases circulation to the brain and stimulates the lymphatic system, which removes toxins and aids digestion. Daily exercise can be revitalizing. People should develop their own exercise routines that work for them.

POSTURE AND ALIGNMENT

Posture and skeletal alignment are also factors in maintaining healthy energy levels. Poor posture and misalignment affect nerve function, and muscle and connective tissue tone, which is essential for optimum energy levels. Yoga is an excellent form of exercise, which has the added value of helping to maintain proper posture. Correcting misalignments with regular chiropractic care can be helpful in achieving good energy levels.

SLEEP

Sufficient and restful sleep is important for maintaining good energy levels. Many people overwork and do not get enough rest. A great deal of repair work occurs during sleep: hormones are manufactured, glands are rejuvenated, and toxins are removed. When people do not get enough sleep, they often use more stimulants to compensate for their insufficient rest. It is important to understand, however, that the body cannot endure long hours of work and overstimulation forever.

Sleep is essential. When we are deprived of it, aging is accelerated and we burn out. Burnout can happen over a long period of time or in a single day. Many people who visit the BioSET clinic say they used to be able to go, go, go and thought nothing could ever happen to slow them down. They felt immune to the physical problems other people had. Overnight, they were suddenly unable to get out of bed, followed by years when they were unable to function well. Other common complaints following a lack of sleep are being unable to work and loss of appetite.

Not everyone needs eight or nine hours of sleep a night, but people know how much rest they need. When you wake up naturally, without an alarm clock, you should have the sleep you need. If you have to use an alarm to wake up, then you may need more sleep or have some imbalances that need to be evaluated.

Some people use sleep aids such as melatonin to help them sleep. However, BioSET practitioners have found that many people are sensitive to melatonin. Released during sleep, melatonin is thought to be an anti-aging and antioxidant chemical. When cleared for melatonin sensitivity, people can use their own melatonin rather than having to take it orally. If there is no sensitivity, the body should be producing enough melatonin and other antioxidants naturally, and there should be no need to take additional melatonin.

MENTAL HEALTH

Mental health, a product of homeostasis and freedom from sensitivities and intolerances, is important for all age groups. When energy levels are low, people are more vulnerable to physical, mental, and emotional problems. When people are tired, they find it difficult to relate, function properly, or conduct business as usual. I know from experience that by strengthening digestion, eliminating sensitivities with digestive enzymes and BioSET clearings, modifying or adjusting the diet, exercising, developing good posture, and practicing meditation and breathing techniques, one can strengthen the body, become more resilient, and reduce the impact of mental and emotional stresses. It is easy to have a positive outlook when one feels rested and energized.

In general, when sensitivities are cleared, digestion and nutrition are improved, and the body is free of toxins and well rested, stable energy levels are fairly easy to maintain. However, some people need extra help in the form of systemic enzyme supplements. These enzyme supplements help to do the following:

+ Fortify the metabolism
+ Improve adrenal function
+ Fight inflammation
+ Promote healing
+ Strengthen the immune system

There are also enzyme formulas especially designed to help sufferers of asthma, sensitivities, and sinus congestion (outlined in chapter 13). BioSET practitioners are fully trained in evaluating when each formula is appropriate. My book *MicroMiracles: Discover the Healing Power of Enzymes* elaborates on these systemic enzyme formulas and their function in healing and well-being.

Energy levels sometimes improve dramatically, but more often they change slowly. After our bodies have been abused for years with coffee, alcohol, and smoking, it may take time to restore adequate energy levels. Even though a double espresso shot with latte can give us some quick energy, it is preferable to allow our energy to rebound slowly by natural means in order to let our bodies heal in their own time. Depression and feelings of anxiety ease as energy levels rise and the body finds its own rhythm. This is evident at any age. Each person must pursue health on every level to maintain abundant energy and vitality throughout their life. Genetics may ensure certain tendencies, but our adherence to natural health will in the end be victorious.

PART FOUR

Adjunctive Therapy

Enzyme Therapy

After many years of working with others, I am delighted to share my own story. At fifty-five, I am healthier now than I was thirty years ago. I owe this feeling of well-being to enzyme therapy, which changed my life, my health, and my practice as a healer and taught me about many miracles of the human body. Above all, it taught me about balance, homeostasis, and how to maintain a healthy digestive and immune system.

My Personal Experience with Enzymes

For as long as I could remember, I suffered from digestive problems. I was constipated, bloated, tired, and depressed. No matter what I ate or when, or how, or with whom I ate it, I would end up feeling like I was three months pregnant. I was bloated constantly, throughout the day. As a result, I always wore loose clothing with an elastic waistband. When I was growing up, both my father and my grandmother had complained of digestive problems, so I assumed it was an inherited condition I would have to live with for the rest of my life.

In the early seventies, I became involved in healing as a profession with an emphasis on massage and polarity therapy. I went on to study homeopathy and nutrition with various doctors, including Dr. Bernard Jensen at his ranch in Escondido. Refusing to believe that my problem and other people's digestive problems were all just inherited, I was determined to find a solution. I studied every book about natural healing available at the time. I tried every vitamin, explored homeopathy, and experimented with many kinds of diets, including fasting. But nothing changed my digestive abnormalities. At times I despaired of ever finding the answer I was seeking.

In 1972 I decided to get a degree in chiropractic. My twin brother had gone into conventional medicine, but I was drawn to a more natural approach. Unlike medical school, chiropractic college offered a good course in diet and nutrition.

During my first year there, probably due to the stress of the coursework, my symptoms worsened. Everything I ate aggravated my digestion, and I became severely constipated and bloated. At the chiropractic clinic affiliated with the school, I received X-rays, barium X-rays, and blood work, and I proceeded to do colonics, fasting, and food rotation. I remember doing a grape fast for almost three months. When I fasted, my symptoms seemed to improve slightly, but I relapsed after I began to eat regular foods. I tried different chiropractic treatments, homeopathy, and other new diets. Again, nothing seemed to help.

After graduating from chiropractic school and practicing for a number of years, I decided to enroll in a three-year postgraduate chiropractic orthopedics training program. This course changed my life, my health, and my professional practice forever because it was there that one of my instructors introduced me to enzymes and enzyme therapy.

When I began to investigate this field, I discovered I was carbohydrate intolerant and that, therefore, I was unable to properly digest and assimilate foods containing sugars and other carbohydrates, including grains and breads. I began taking an enzyme consisting of disaccharridase, cellulase, maltase, sucrase, and lactase to help me digest sugars and carbohydrates. Two weeks after beginning the enzymes, the bloating and constipation I had experienced my whole life disappeared and have never returned. It was miraculous.

After this total regeneration of my digestive system, I studied enzymes and enzyme therapy extensively and began to utilize enzyme therapy in my practice. I also noticed other changes in my health. I had more energy, my hair and nails were healthier, I needed less sleep, and my immune system was considerably healthier. So I decided that with each individual patient, I would recommend an enzyme protocol, along with a diet based on their specific food intolerances. These diets, along with a comprehensive overview of the role enzymes play in health and longevity, are presented in *MicroMiracles: Discover the Healing Power of Enzymes.*

After careful study and trial and error, I finally developed the best diet for myself, what I call the carbohydrate-intolerant diet. This is a very important food program because I have found that 80–90 percent of the people who come to see BioSET practitioners are carbohydrate intolerant. Aside from bloating and constipation, sugar intolerance can lead to diabetes, adrenal dysfunction, asthma, hyperactivity, attention deficit disorder, depression, fatigue, poor assimilation of foods, obesity, or malnutrition, and frequent sore throats, ear infections, and colds. It can also be responsible for chronic yeast infections and chronic food and environmental sensitivities. I suffered from many of these problems myself, and the carbohydrate-intolerant diet I developed has changed my life. This diet is low in carbohydrates (no grains permitted), fruits, and sweet vegetables and high in protein. There is a version that incorporates vegetable protein for vegetarians. I myself am a vegan and eat as much of my food raw as possible. I recommend this diet for all carbohydrate-intolerant people.

My regeneration occurred about twenty-five years ago. I am so enthusiastic about enzyme support that my family, colleagues, and patients jokingly call me the Enzyme Empress. Since they've seen what enzymes have done for me, everyone I know is now taking enzymes. They can change your health forever.

What Are Enzymes?

Enzymes are complex proteins in the body that accelerate chemical changes in other substances in order to provide the labor force and energy necessary to keep us alive. They are energy catalysts that are essential for the successful occurrence of over 150,000 biochemical reactions in our bodies, particularly those involving food digestion and the delivery of nutrients to the body. Enzymes help convert food into chemical substances that can pass into cell membranes to perform all of our everyday life-sustaining functions. By supporting normal function, enzymes keep our immune systems strong enough to fight off disease. Enzymes help to nourish and clean the body, making possible the human body's miraculous capacity for self-healing. Enzymes also make available the energy needed for a normal body to burn hundreds of grams of carbohydrates and fat every day. Without enzymes, life could not be sustained.

Enzymes perform so many important functions in the body that they have been called the basis of all systemic activity. Some of the various enzymes' responsibilities include the following:

+ Transforming foods into muscles, nerves, bones, and glands
+ Helping to store excess foods in muscles or the liver for future use
+ Helping to pass carbon dioxide from the lungs
+ Metabolizing iron for use by the blood
+ Aiding in blood coagulation

- Decomposing hydrogen peroxide and liberating healthful oxygen
- Attacking toxic substances in the body so they can be eliminated, which is essential for patients with chronic health problems
- Helping convert dietary phosphorus to bone
- Extracting minerals from food for use
- Converting protein, carbohydrates, fats, vitamins, and nutrients for the body's use

In other words, enzymes deliver nutrients, break down and carry away toxic waste, digest food, purify the blood, deliver hormones, balance cholesterol and triglyceride levels, feed the brain, build protein into muscle, and feed and fortify the endocrine system. Enzymes also contribute to immune system activity; white blood cells are especially enzyme rich, enabling them to digest foreign invading substances.

OUR ENZYME POTENTIAL

While one of the advantages of enzymes is that they can cause a chemical reaction without being destroyed or changed in the process, the number of enzymes we can produce in a lifetime is limited. Every person is born with an enzyme potential (the number of enzymes he or she can produce in a lifetime), which is determined by their DNA code. In addition, each enzyme can only perform a certain amount of work before it becomes exhausted and must be replaced by another.

Things that diminish a person's available enzyme supply include the following:

- Digesting processed food (assimilating these foods is hard on the body)
- Drinking caffeinated and alcoholic beverages
- Colds and fevers
- Pregnancy
- Stress
- Strenuous exercise
- Injuries
- Extreme weather conditions

If we do not eat an enzyme-rich diet, we deplete our enzyme potential without replenishing it. This is why supplementation and a good diet are essential. When all enzyme activity stops, the body stops functioning and the person dies. However, humans have the capacity to store external food enzymes to ensure the body's ability to metabolize the needed nutrients. This explains the popularity and abundance of new enzyme health products and the recommendations from experts that people supplement their diet with raw foods and enzyme supplements. Many industries have also used enzymes in various products and processes, including laundry detergents, skin care, meat tenderizers, agricultural processes, and waste conversion.

Enzymes can save people's lives by restoring energy and homeostasis, reversing the aging process, turning a dysfunctional digestive system into a healthy one, and strengthening the immune system. In my fifteen years of working with enzyme therapy, I have witnessed enormous success with a variety of illnesses, and the most noticeable and immediate change in each case has always been in the energy level. Patients no longer feel that crash after meals, especially at the most common time, right after lunch.

COENZYMES

Coenzyme Q10 (CoQ10) is important for all the cells in the body to produce energy. Coenzymes help activate enzymes. For example, copper, iron, and other minerals and vitamins, including the B complex, are coenzymes. We need to absorb those important vitamins from our foods so our enzymes and coenzymes can function optimally. Coenzyme Q10, which occurs naturally in the body, has been found useful for heart problems, high blood pressure, asthma,[1] diabetes, cancer, obesity, tumors, and candida. Athletes take CoQ10 for increased endurance.

Why Do We Need Enzymes?

Simply put, enzymes enable our bodies to digest the food we eat. They break down the various foods we consume—proteins, fats, carbohydrates, and vitamins—into smaller compounds that the body can absorb. They are absolutely essential in maintaining optimal health.

Enzymes are present naturally in raw foods, but they are destroyed during the cooking process. For this reason, it is important to eat as much raw food as possible, to subject food to as little heating as possible, and to chew food well, because enzyme production begins in the mouth. Human saliva contains the necessary factors needed to activate plant enzymes in the food we eat, but we need to chew each mouthful extremely well for complete predigestion. Because we often fail to follow these guidelines, we do not receive all the enzymes we need to do the job of digestion. Enzyme supplements provide the missing pieces. Maintaining the body's enzyme levels is critical today, when so much of the food in a typical American diet is processed or cooked. Enzymes are only found naturally in raw foods such as vegetables and fruits, which contain the very enzymes needed to digest them. Food enzymes are extremely heat sensitive, especially at or above temperatures of 118 degrees Fahrenheit. When raw foods are processed or heated in any way (steamed, baked, boiled, stewed, fried, microwaved, or canned), they may lose 100 percent of their enzyme activity and up to 85 percent of their vitamin and mineral content. Even the raw food we eat could be enzyme deficient if it was grown in soils lacking in nutrients. In addition, enzyme deterioration begins the moment food is picked or killed. For all these reasons, supplementing with enzymes is crucial to achieve a more efficient digestive process and better utilization of our food's nutrients.

When digestion is not completed properly, partially digested proteins putrefy, partially digested carbohydrates ferment, partially digested fats turn rancid, and these toxins remain in the body, harming the system. Fermented toxins in the digestive tract may be absorbed into the blood and deposited as waste in the joints and other soft-tissue areas.

The results of enzyme deficiency can include digestive disturbance, fatigue, headaches, constipation, gas, heartburn, bloating, colon problems, excess body fat, and problems as serious as cardiovascular or heart disease. Enzyme deficiencies have been linked to premature aging and degenerative diseases as well. Cancer research has discovered that certain enzymes are completely lacking in the blood and urine of cancer patients. Research has also shown that the body increases white blood cell levels to compensate for an enzyme-deficient diet. Having to use the immune system to aid in digestion whenever enzymes are lacking compromises the body's ability to defend itself from disease.

Digestion has first priority for the limited number of internal enzymes available; systemic enzymes must be satisfied with whatever is left. When we eat food that is devoid of enzymes, the body must draw on its own internal supply of enzymes, both systemic and digestive. Eventually, we deplete our limited reserves, forcing the immune system to aid in digestion instead of rebuilding the body and fighting illness. The pancreas, salivary glands, stomach, and intestines all might contribute the enzymes needed for digestion, robbing the body of systemic enzymes needed for muscles, nerves, blood, and other glands.

When food enzymes are introduced from outside the body, the body does not need to manufacture as many digestive enzymes, allocating more of our enzyme potential toward the production of the systemic enzymes we need for growth, maintenance, and repair.

Enzyme supplements help create more energy, promote faster and easier digestion, and encourage superior nutrient absorption. It is our digestive system's responsibility to release the nutrients that are trapped in our food by breaking the food down. But our digestive system works best when enzyme supplements assist in setting the nutrients free for the body to absorb and use. Receiving all the nutrients in the food we eat is critical since these nutrients are needed to build and repair the body's tissue, produce energy, and maintain a strong immune system.

In the BioSET clinic and institute, we see many patients with chronic food intolerances. For example, people can inherit or develop intolerances to proteins, sugars, fibers, complex carbohydrates, or fats. These patients lack the enzymes they need to break down the food that causes them trouble. Through muscle or electronic testing, BioSET practitioners are able to ascertain which foods a person cannot tolerate and which enzymes they need to supplement with to restore proper digestion and food tolerance. With the proper enzyme supplements, these patients regain the ability to digest their food properly and thoroughly.

PROTEIN INTOLERANCE

People who do not digest proteins crave them. They tend to experience anxiety, osteoporosis, edema, eye or ear inflammation, endometriosis, and bone spurs.

Carla, a fifty-year-old patient, had a family history of osteoporosis and arthritis. She also complained of bloating and indigestion. Two years earlier she had been screened for osteoporosis, and the results suggested that she might have already developed the disease. She was advised to eat dairy products and to take 1,500 mg of calcium daily. After two years she was tested again, and the results were even worse.

Worried, upset, and afraid, she came to me for a nutritional consultation. When I performed an enzyme evaluation, the results showed that she was deficient in calcium and sensitive to her calcium supplements and the dairy products she had been eating. After prescribing a carbohydrate digestive enzyme to help ease her dairy sensitivity, I also cleared her for calcium and prescribed a mineral enzyme formula. In one year, her test results were significantly better. I often wonder how many of the millions of women who take calcium supplements to prevent osteoporosis and arthritis are sensitive to the very thing to which they are overloading their bodies.

SUGAR INTOLERANCE

People who are sugar intolerant tend to crave sugar and often suffer from depression, malabsorption of nutrients, bloating, food sensitivities, hyperactivity, Crohn's disease or colitis, asthma, chronic ear infections, and constipation.

CARBOHYDRATE INTOLERANCE

Carbohydrate intolerance affects most of the population and definitely describes the asthmatic.

FAT INTOLERANCE

People who are fat intolerant tend to crave fat and salt, and they often suffer from eczema, liver and gallbladder disease, and toxicity.

Types of Enzymes

There are three main categories of enzymes: systemic, digestive, and food.

SYSTEMIC ENZYMES

Systemic enzymes are produced internally and are responsible for managing and regulating all processes in the body that have to do with the blood, tissues, and organs. They are required for the growth of new cells and the repair and maintenance of all the body's organs and tissues. Systemic enzymes take protein, fat, and carbohydrates and transform them into the proper balance of working cells and tissues. Systemic enzymes also remove worn-out material from the cells, keeping them clean and healthy.

DIGESTIVE ENZYMES

Digestive enzymes are also produced internally and deal with the digestion of food and the absorption and delivery of nutrients throughout the body. The most commonly known digestive enzymes are secreted from the pancreas into the stomach and small intestine. Each enzyme is specific to a particular compound, which it can break down or synthesize. The three most important enzymes for digestion are protease (digests protein), amylase (digests carbohydrates), and lipase (digests fat).

FOOD ENZYMES

Food enzymes, the only enzymes that are produced externally, are derived solely from raw fruits, vegetables, and supplemental sources. They help the digestive enzymes break down food. Food enzymes need vitamins and minerals, called cofactors, to be present for proper functioning. Unlike raw enzymes, cofactors are not completely destroyed by cooking. But since raw food enzymes become useless after heat processing, the cofactors in our diet are not utilized to their full potential.

Enzymes perform their best at a certain pH level. For example, animal enzymes perform best at a pH of 6.5–9.0. On the other hand, vegetarian enzymes have a broader pH range. I prefer to use full-spectrum vegetarian enzymes because they can survive transport through the stomach's acidic pH (pH 2.0) and can be used in the pancreas and small intestine to further digestion.

Some of the reported benefits of consuming vegetarian digestive enzymes include the elimination of the following:

+ Heartburn
+ Gas
+ Headaches
+ Bloating
+ Colon problems
+ Stress
+ Fatigue after meals
+ Problems with being overweight and underweight
+ Constipation or loose bowels
+ Weakened immune system
+ Food sensitivities
+ Hay fever

The conventional wisdom among physicians and nutritionists is that food enzymes are destroyed once food hits the stomach, because the food sits in acid for at least thirty minutes. In fact, there's a time lag between this phase of digestion and the one preceding it. As food leaves the esophagus, it drops into the top portion of the stomach, which has very little acid, and remains there for thirty to forty-five minutes before moving on. All the while, the enzymes continue doing their job. Even when the food moves to the bottom portion of the stomach, the enzymes remain active until the acid level becomes prohibitive. Then a special acid enzyme, pepsin, can continue the digestion of protein where the other enzymes left off.

How do we know all this? Researchers have gained this information by pumping out and examining the contents of the stomach and upper intestinal contents at various intervals following meals.

The Primary Digestive Enzymes

The following are the main digestive enzymes that are used therapeutically to help restore the body's homeostasis and strengthen the immune system.

PROTEASE:

+ Breaks down protein
+ Acts on pathogens such as bacteria, viruses, and even cancer cells
+ Breaks down protein into amino acids
+ Works best in the high acidity of the stomach
+ Is also found in pancreatic and intestinal juices

AMYLASE:

+ Breaks down carbohydrates (starches) into simpler sugars such as dextrin and maltose
+ Is found in our saliva, pancreas, and intestines
+ Is secreted by the salivary glands and the pancreas

LIPASE:

+ Along with bile from the gallbladder, breaks down fats and the oil-soluble vitamins A, D, E, and F
+ Is helpful for weight loss and for cardiovascular conditions
+ Splits fats into glycerol and fatty acids

CELLULASE:

+ Breaks down fiber and cellulose (found in fruits, vegetables, grains, seeds, and plant material)

+ Can increase the nutritional value of fruits and vegetables
+ Prevents putrefaction, bloating, and gas; foods high in cellulose must be chewed well for it to work

PECTINASE:

+ Breaks down pectin-rich foods such as citrus fruits, apples, carrots, potatoes, beets, and tomatoes

LACTASE:

+ Breaks down lactose, the complex sugar in milk products
+ Is ideal for lactose-intolerant individuals
+ Is usually produced in smaller quantities with age

CATHEPSIN:

+ Breaks down meat from animals

ANTIOXIDANT ENZYME:

+ Protects us from the negative effects of free radicals, highly reactive compounds that can damage almost any cell in the body

BROMELAIN:

+ Breaks down food protein into smaller peptones by hydrolysis
+ Can help the body to fight cancer, improve circulation, and treat inflammation (after a musculoskeletal injury it can reduce inflammation as well as, or even better than, any anti-inflammatory drug)
+ Is said to improve the effect of some antibiotics
+ Assists absorption of nutrients from foods and supplements
+ Reduces swelling after dental surgery
+ Helps in dysmenorrhea (painful periods)
+ Increases tissue permeability
+ Can prevent the narrowing of arteries, which contributes to heart attacks

PAPAIN:

+ Breaks down food protein into smaller peptones by hydrolysis
+ Aids the body in digestion

GLUCOAMYLASE:

+ Breaks down maltose (the sugar in all grains that may cause cravings for breads and carbohydrates) into two glucose molecules, allowing greater absorption of this energy-giving sugar

INVERTASE:

+ Helps the body to assimilate and utilize sucrose, a sugar that can contribute to digestive stress if not properly digested

Some herbs also aid digestion, such as aloe vera, which provides relief from peptic ulcers and helps with constipation, and slippery elm, which is good for hiatal hernias and acid reflux, both common symptoms in asthmatics.

Therapeutic Use of Enzyme Supplements with Asthma

According to Hippocrates, "Man is not nourished by what he swallows, but by what he digests and uses." With the increasing pollution and depletion of healthy soil, the foods we eat today have only a fraction of the nutrition our ancestors might have consumed in centuries past. At the same time, we now have the advanced technology that allows us to replenish the nutrients we lose through food processing by taking enzyme supplements with every meal.

Once known only to alternative health professionals, enzyme therapy has achieved such amazing results (measured by patient evaluations as well as by microscopic blood analysis) that the treatment has recently excited even the medical mainstream.

Enzymes can provide relief for asthmatics and people with sensitivities and sinus congestion. One of the most common complaints I hear from the asthmatics I see in my practice is "I don't have enough energy." For the most part, low energy occurs because people are not digesting their food properly and, therefore, cannot benefit from the energy that food can provide. Instead of deriving the needed enzymes directly from the food itself, the body has to borrow enzymes from its metabolism, which requires energy. In fact, digesting food without an adequate amount of enzymes can actually use up more energy than the food can provide. Reversing this situation frees up the body's energy for other tasks.

The regular consumption of enzyme supplements brings numerous positive benefits in terms of ongoing general health, including the following:

+ The prevention of toxic waste buildup in the intestines
+ More efficient assimilation of fats and proteins in the body
+ More comfortable, efficient absorption of nutrients
+ More comfortable digestion of large amounts of carbohydrates
+ An accelerated digestive process due to catalyzation from enzymes

According to Dr. Edward Howell, who researched the effect of enzymes for more than fifty years, it is extremely possible that every degenerative disease, including asthma, may have its origin in a raw food enzyme deficiency. In response to this research, enzyme advocate William E. Frazier remarked, "Not to realize that most, if not all, degenerative diseases are traceable to a common denominator, and that common denominator being the food that we eat for nourishment, is an insult to human intelligence."

ENERGY AND DIGESTIVE ENZYMES

After a large meal, you may notice a sudden feeling of sluggishness and energy loss. Your body is faced with an overload of calories and nutrients to break down and deliver to the bloodstream. If the food you ate was cooked, there are no longer any enzymes in it to assist in the energy-consuming task of digestion. If an enzyme supplement is taken at the beginning of a meal, the body is armed and prepared to handle the new food entering the digestive system. Without this additional supply of enzymes ready, it may take the body up to sixty minutes to gather the needed enzymes, sometimes borrowing them from other systemic processes. When supplemental food enzymes are used, time and energy are conserved, allowing for more complete absorption of nutrients from the food consumed. When food enzymes are taken between meals as well, they are absorbed into the bloodstream and distributed throughout the body rather than being used for digestion.

THE IMMUNE SYSTEM

Systemic enzymes play a vital role in building and strengthening a healthy immune system, which is one of the major goals when working with asthmatics. A strong immune system enables a body to be less vulnerable to viruses, bacteria, parasites, and other toxic invaders. It also helps the body stay healthy during times of stress and when a complete and balanced diet is not followed. Systemic enzyme supplements help to ensure that an asthmatic's immune system is in good condition.

CIRCULATING IMMUNE COMPLEXES (CICS) AND DIGESTIVE ENZYMES

When substantial amounts of food remain undigested, these undigested food residues seep into the bloodstream. There they are viewed as antigens and quickly become attached to tiny antibodies, forming antigen-antibody complexes known as circulating immune complexes (CICs). These tiny immune complexes float freely in the blood or the lymph until they are gobbled up by the large macrophages, the Pacmen of the body.

But if the macrophages overlook the CICs, or if chemotherapeutic drugs, steroids, or excessive antibiotics suppress the macrophages, the CICs can grow in size and latch themselves onto body tissue. Then the backup immune defense system (T and B cells, produced by the bone marrow) starts destroying its own tissue cells in an attempt to destroy these CICs. Unfortunately, the body's noble effort generally backfires and an inflammatory immune response may occur, creating inflammation, redness, and swelling. Glomerulonephritis (a kidney disease), colitis, arthritis, fibromyalgia, migraines, and asthma are conditions that may be aggravated or worsened by this response. Certain enzymes, especially protease, can break up these CICs and reduce inflammation. Asthmatics should take protease regularly, so the immune system is enhanced and can better protect the individual by fighting off infections. With enzyme supplementation, there is an immediate decrease in chronic bacterial infection and inflammation.

INFLAMMATION AND SYSTEMIC ENZYMES

Inflammation, or swelling, is a body's normal response to injury or infection. The first phase of the inflammation process is the body's fight against the infection, the second is repairing the damaged tissue, and the third is cleaning up debris and dead tissue. White blood cells circulate throughout the blood and lymph all the time. During the dynamic process of inflammation and repair, there is increased blood flow to the area, causing blood clots and obstructing blood flow, which in turn causes swelling and oozing. A barrier of fibrin is formed to encircle the area of inflammation. The healing process then begins to occur.

Usually, when the healing is complete, the inflammation subsides. Sometimes the healing process causes scarring. The central issue in asthma, however, is that often the inflammation does not resolve completely on its own. In the short term, this results in recurrent asthma attacks. In the long term, it may lead to a permanent thickening of the bronchial walls, called airway "remodeling." If the bronchial tubes narrow, this may become irreversible. Therefore, controlling airway inflammation in order to reduce the reactivity of the airways can prevent airway remodeling.

Both acute and chronic inflammation can be greatly helped with the use of systemic enzymes. Systemic enzymes, such as protease and amylase, can help bring more oxygen to the area and reduce swelling by breaking up the fibrous tissue and eating up the dead and infected tissue. This in turn speeds healing and reduces pain. Enzymes can remove foreign bodies, such as bacteria, viruses, and other microorganisms, and they can help to clean up the area so that new nerve tissue and cells can be formed.

Taking protease and amylase in combination with other herbal extracts (see enzyme listings later in the chapter) can serve to significantly reduce inflammation in asthmatics. Enzymes, by restoring digestion, cleansing an area, and preventing inflammation, can be very beneficial to asthmatics and all individuals with sensitivities. In conventional medicine, cortisone therapy is often used to treat chronic inflammatory problems, such as Crohn's disease. Cortisone can help stop inflammation in the short run, but in the long run it can make a situation worse because it blocks the body's natural immune function. The bacteria, parasite, fungus, or other pathogens that cause the irritation can continue to destroy and invade the body, as the immune system remains paralyzed by the cortisone, unable to fight. Even though the inflammation is curtailed, the pathogenic process still prevails and may even worsen, causing more irritation and other autoimmune problems.

Unlike cortisone, enzymes do not inhibit the immune system, instead promoting the healing process by attacking pathogens and, ultimately, reducing swelling and inflammation. Enzyme preparations can be used to support a wide variety of chronic inflammatory conditions, including bronchitis, asthma, rheumatoid arthritis, sinusitis, kidney infections, ear infections, herpes zoster, and outbreaks of herpes simplex 1 and 2.

THE IMMUNE SYSTEM AND ANTIOXIDANTS PLUS DIGESTIVE ENZYMES

BioSET practitioners use antioxidant supplements and enzyme therapy to strengthen the immune systems of asthmatics. Children with asthma are usually sugar intolerant, which is not surprising given that the annual sugar consumption in the United States is now 150 pounds per capita. In fact, recent studies indicate that 80 percent of the population is sugar intolerant. This intolerance involves all sugars, including fruit, grains, and artificial sugars, such as sorbitol, Equal, Nutrasweet, Splenda, and mannitol.

Those who suffer from asthma frequently have B vitamin deficiencies, which can be caused by an overabundance of sugar. Asthmatics also tend to be sensitive to B vitamins, which may contribute to the deficiency. Other dietary intolerances that aggravate asthma include food additives, sodium metabisulfites, and excessive consumption of protein, which creates an acid situation in the body.

Overconsumption and underdigestion of protein can add to the excess acidity that respiratory distress causes in asthmatics. Hypothyroid, hypoadrenal, and chronic intestinal toxemia can also contribute to asthma. Most asthmatics will benefit from an enzyme that contains the four food enzymes plus three disaccharidases—sucrase, lactase, and maltase—and a respiratory enzyme formula containing enzymes and herbs that nourish the lungs, help expectorate mucus, and relieve coughing and wheezing.

ENVIRONMENTAL TOXINS AND DIGESTIVE ENZYMES

Toxins in our environment, chemotherapy treatment, radiation, and unhealthy lifestyles all contribute to the breakdown of the immune system. Enzymes can interrupt the damage and inflammation that go along with these stresses to the immune system, which will benefit the asthmatic individual.

Millions of people take vitamin, mineral, and protein supplements, but they may be a waste of money unless you have sufficient enzymes to help digest and absorb these nutrients. The body requires air, water, proteins, carbohydrates, vitamins, good fats, minerals, and enzymes, and no one nutrient can properly function if any of the others is deficient. Enzymes and their coworkers—minerals, vitamins, protein, water, fats, and carbohydrates—are all essential. Enzymes destroy toxins, free radicals, and antigens in the liver and bloodstream.

SENSITIVITIES AND DIGESTIVE ENZYMES

Many of people's sensitivities today are actually related to a lack of certain enzymes needed to digest the substance that causes their sensitivity reaction. Joint pain and gout often result from undigested proteins, fats, and minerals, which form uric crystals that get caught in the joints. Yeast and fungal growth can start with undigested foods in the bloodstream and may be compounded by the white flour and sugar we eat. Extreme fatigue may be a consequence of an inability to digest proteins and fats, which causes poor circulation. When blood clumps together, it cannot carry as much oxygen, which can lead to slow and muddled thinking. It is also more difficult for white blood cells to travel where they are needed when they are caught in sluggish, clumped blood.

Proteolytic and lipolytic enzymes found in some supplements help to break down unwanted toxins and irritants that can be partially responsible for sensitivities and inflammation. The enzymes break the toxic substances into smaller, more manageable components that the body can then eliminate.

THE IMMUNE SYSTEM AND ANTIOXIDANTS

Superoxide dismutase (SOD), a copper- and zinc-containing enzyme found in all body cells, is a primary defender against free radicals. Reactive oxygen molecules, or oxygen radicals, can destroy healthy tissue. SOD eliminates destructive superoxide molecules, common free radicals produced in the body, and soaks up free radical oxygen molecules in the bloodstream.

Normally, the body makes enough SOD to hold oxygen radicals in check. But when the immune system gets ready to destroy bacteria or other infectants or invaders, the surge in the number of white blood cells or antibodies triggers a rapid proliferation of oxygen radicals. In many inflammatory conditions such as asthma, the white blood cells or immune reactors identify certain tissues as foreign and begin to attack them. SOD can scavenge the free radicals and interrupt the progress of this inflammatory reaction.

SOD also inhibits fats in the cells from becoming rancid, which can help prevent premature aging. It also helps wounds to heal and alleviates symptoms related to radiation sickness. Some people are deficient in this enzyme and may need to use a supplement. The food sources of SOD are green vegetables, yeast, sprouted seeds, and grains.

Dr. Ellen's Enzyme Recommendations

Enzymes are specific supplements with natural ingredients for digestion and systemic purposes. The following products provide potent enzyme blends. Enzymes are measured in units that measure their levels of activity, such as DU, MU, and HUT.

ADRENAL HEALTH

Stress is a part of everyday life, and the adrenal glands play a key role in regulating your mental and physical responses. Prolonged stress exhausts the adrenals, resulting in fatigue, irritability, and a lowered immune response, among other symptoms. Adrenal Health supports the adrenals and boosts their stress-resisting capabilities to improve mental and physical stamina and restore vitality and well-being.

Two vegetarian capsules of Adrenal Health taken twice per day on an empty stomach provide the following:

Anti-stress herbs:

+ Panax ginseng root extract (standardized to contain 8 percent ginsenosides)—160 mg
+ Bupleurum root extract—100 mg (equivalent to 400 mg of raw herb)
+ Rice bran (a source of B vitamins)—65 mg
+ Siberian ginseng root extract (standardized to contain 0.8 percent eleutherosides)—40 mg

Adrenal Health:

+ pHysioProtease—30,000 HUT (177,600 pHysio-U)
+ CereCalase Plus—100 MU

COLON HEALTH

The friendly bacteria that normally live in the colon play a vital role in health. Colon Health provides a blend of over three billion viable probiotic organisms to restore the colon's flora balance, which can be disrupted by illness or gastrointestinal disturbances. These organisms impede the growth of harmful bacteria, viruses, fungi, and yeast and raise the colon's pH to help inhibit potentially harmful tissue changes. They also increase the body's natural supply of lactase to overcome lactose intolerance.

One vegetarian capsule of Colon Health taken one or two times per day, preferably upon arising or at bedtime, provides the following:

Health-promoting probiotics:

+ Lactobacillus acidophilus—1 billion organisms
+ Lactobacillus plantarum—1 billion organisms
+ Bifidobacterium bifidum—500 million organisms
+ Lactobacillus salivarius—250 million organisms
+ Lactobacillus casei—250 million organisms

DIGESTIVE HEALTH

Proper digestion is essential to maintaining wellness. Digestive Health provides a superior blend of eighteen different enzymes to aid in digesting every component of your food. Take one or more capsules with every meal or snack to enhance digestion and to release all of your food's nutrients. Improved digestion can almost immediately reduce the bloating, belching, gas, indigestion, and fatigue that often accompany a meal. Over time, supplemental digestive enzymes increase your overall energy level because your body needs less energy for digestion. As you get more from your food, your appetite may also decrease.

One vegetarian capsule of Digestive Health taken with each meal provides the following:

Protein-digesting enzymes:

+ Protease blend (alkaline, neutral, and acid proteases plus peptidase)— 25,000 HUT

Fat-digesting enzymes:

+ Lipase—200 LU

Sugar-digesting enzymes:

+ Invertase—375 SU (0.75 IAU)
+ Lactase—200 ALU/LacU
+ Alpha-galactosidase—20 GalU (50 AGSU)

Starch-digesting enzymes:

+ Amylase—10,000 DU
+ Glucoamylase—14 AGU
+ Malt diastase—375 DP°

Fiber-digesting enzymes:

+ Cellulase—450 CU
+ CereCalase Plus—50 MU
+ Xylanase—100 XU
+ Pectinase—2 endo-PGU

DIGESTIVE CHEWABLES

Natural raspberry-flavored chewable tablets, Digestive Chewables provide all the enzymes needed to digest protein, carbohydrates, fat, and fiber in your food. These are ideal for people who have difficulty swallowing capsules or who just prefer a supplement that tastes good.

One Digestive Chewable vegetarian tablet taken with each meal provides the following:

Protein-digesting enzymes:

+ Protease blend (alkaline, neutral, and acid proteases plus peptidase)— 20,000 HUT

Fat-digesting enzymes:

+ Lipase—200 LU

Sugar-digesting enzymes:

+ Invertase—375 SU (0.75 IAU)
+ Lactase—500 ALU/LacU
+ Alpha-galactosidase—10 GalU (25 AGSU)

Starch-digesting enzymes:

+ Amylase—7,000 DU
+ Glucoamylase—15 AGU
+ Malt diastase—250 DP°

Fiber-digesting enzymes:

+ Cellulase—300 CU
+ CereCalase—50 MU
+ Pectinase—5 endo-PGU

Other ingredients:

Dextrose (corn sugar), fructose (fruit sugar), natural raspberry flavor, silica (mineral), plant cellulose, citric acid, vegetarian magnesium stearate, and proprietary plant-derived sweetener.

GASTRIC EASE

Chronic nausea or abdominal discomfort may indicate damage to the lining of the gastrointestinal tract, resulting in incomplete digestion and nutritional deficiencies. Gastric Ease helps soothe and protect the gastrointestinal lining and promotes thorough digestion when taken with meals. The body can then utilize all of your food's nutrients to help repair and maintain a healthy gut. Take Gastric Ease between meals instead of an antacid at the next sign of gastric distress.

One vegetarian capsule of Gastric Ease taken with each meal or between meals as needed provides the following:

Soothing herbs:

+ Marshmallow root—85 mg
+ Marshmallow root extract—50 mg (equivalent to 200 mg of raw herb)
+ Aloe vera gel extract—10 mg (equivalent to 2,000 mg of raw gel)

Protein-digesting enzymes:

+ Peptidase—1,000 HUT

Fat-digesting enzymes:

+ Lipase—150 LU

Sugar-digesting enzymes:

+ Invertase—100 SU (0.2 IAU)
+ Lactase—75 ALU/LacU
+ Alpha-galactosidase—10 GalU (25 AGSU)

Starch-digesting enzymes:

+ Amylase—3,000 DU
+ Glucoamylase—4 AGU
+ Malt diastase—100 DP°

Fiber-digesting enzymes:

+ Cellulase—200 CU
+ CereCalase Plus—50 MU
+ Xylanase—50 XU
+ Pectinase—1 endo-PGU

KIDNEY/BLADDER HEALTH

The kidneys and bladder play an important role in eliminating wastes from the body and regulating electrolytes in the blood. Kidney/Bladder Health helps maintain the integrity of urinary tract tissue, strengthen the body's defenses against harmful bacteria in the urinary tract, and promote the excretion of urine.

Two vegetarian capsules of Kidney/Bladder Health taken twice per day on an empty stomach provide the following:

Antiseptic herbs:

+ Uva ursi leaf extract (standardized to contain 20 percent arbutin)— 200 mg
+ Corn silk extract (equivalent to 320 mg of raw herb)—80 mg
+ Goldenseal root extract (standardized to contain 5 percent total alkaloids)—60 mg

Natural-source vitamin:

+ Vitamin A (beta-carotene from Dunaliella algae)—4,000 IU

Enzymes:

+ pHysioProtease—40,000 HUT (236,800 pHysio-U)

LUNG HEALTH

The lungs exchange life-giving oxygen for carbon dioxide, and their cleansing mechanism uses fluid mucus to keep dust, organisms, and other irritants out of the lungs. Lung Health strengthens the respiratory tract's own natural defenses by protecting and soothing the lungs' lining and helping to keep air passages open, making breathing easier. It also stimulates mucus production while enabling rapid clearing of mucus from the lungs.

Two vegetarian Lung Health capsules taken twice per day on an empty stomach provide the following:

Protective herbs:

+ Thyme herb extract—130 mg (equivalent to 520 mg of raw herb)
+ Mullein leaf extract—100 mg (equivalent to 400 mg of raw herb)
+ Great plantain leaf extract—40 mg (equivalent to 160 mg of raw herb)

- Acerola cherries extract (standardized to contain 17 percent vitamin C)—40 mg
- Quercetin—20 mg
- Rice bran (a source of B vitamins)—20 mg

Enzymes:

- pHysioProtease—36,000 HUT (213,120 pHysio-U)
- Amylase—1,000 DU
- CereCalase Plus—40 MU

NASAL CLEAR

Common upper respiratory symptoms such as nasal and sinus congestion, sneezing, itchy eyes, and discomfort in the ears or throat result from a weakened immune system. Nasal Clear, when taken for a few months before and during the high pollen season, helps to strengthen a body's natural resistance to harmful microorganisms and other airborne irritants, normalize mucus production, tone the membranes of the upper respiratory tract, and control the release of natural inflammatory substances.

Three vegetarian Nasal Clear capsules taken once per day on an empty stomach provide the following:

Decongesting herbs:

- Elder flower extract—150 mg (equivalent to 600 mg of raw herb)
- *Echinacea purpurea/Echinacea angustifolia* root extract—150 mg (equivalent to 600 mg of raw herb)
- Acerola cherries extract (standardized to contain 17 percent vitamin C)—60 mg
- Quercetin—45 mg
- Eyebright herb extract—45 mg (equivalent to 180 mg of raw herb)
- Goldenseal root extract (standardized to contain 5 percent total alkaloids)—30 mg
- Rice bran (a source of B vitamins)—30 mg

Bioavailable mineral:

- Zinc (from zinc citrate)—9 mg

Enzymes:

- ✦ pHysioProtease—43,500 HUT (257,520 pHysio-U)
- ✦ Peptidase—1,500 HUT
- ✦ Amylase—3,000 DU
- ✦ CereCalase Plus—60 MU

PROTEASE

A healthy body uses its own protease enzymes to normalize inflammation, detoxify the blood, maintain a strong immune system, regulate hormones, and speed tissue repair. Taking Protease, the supplement, between meals on an empty stomach ensures that adequate quantities of protease will always be available for these important functions. Protease provides pHysioProtease, a proprietary blend of proteases proven through independent research to be the only protease blend available that is optimally active in blood and body tissues.

One vegetarian capsule of Protease taken two to three times per day on an empty stomach provides the following:

Potent enzymes:

- ✦ pHysioProtease—200,000 HUT (1,184,000 pHysio-U)

Bioavailable mineral:

- ✦ Calcium (from calcium citrate)—20 mg

SLEEP ENHANCE

Everyone suffers from sleep disturbances at one time or another. Whether it's difficulty falling asleep or frequent awakenings during the night, loss of sleep impairs your ability to function during the day. Sleep Enhance is a safe, nonaddictive sleep aid that promotes restful sleep by normalizing sleep patterns, without causing daytime drowsiness. It helps to hasten the onset of sleep, eliminate nighttime awakenings, and improve sleep quality, thereby enhancing overall well-being.

Two vegetarian capsules of Sleep Enhance taken thirty minutes prior to bedtime provide the following:

Resting herbs:

+ Valerian root extract—200 mg (equivalent to 800 mg of raw herb)
+ Passionflower herb extract—120 mg (equivalent to 480 mg of raw herb)
+ Wild lettuce leaf extract—40 mg (equivalent to 160 mg of raw herb)
+ Oat straw extract—30 mg (equivalent to 300 mg of raw herb)
+ Rice bran (a source of B vitamins)—20 mg

Enzymes:

+ pHysioProtease—16,000 HUT (94,720 pHysio-U)
+ CereCalase Plus—40 MU

PART FIVE

Case Studies

BioSET and Enzyme Case Studies

The following case histories examine instances where enzymes were crucial in the healing process for individuals with asthma.

Infectants: Fungu—Mold and Mildew

In this case history, mold and fungus were the underlying triggers for the symptoms.

Case 1: Leslie

Leslie, a five-year-old girl who had suffered from severe asthma since birth, came to see me with Jane, her mother. Jane was frustrated, distressed, and frightened about her daughter's health. The day they came to see me, Leslie had been given a variety of medications, including antibiotics, steroids, cough syrup, and inhalers. Her mother explained that she was not herself because the medications caused severe mood swings, behavioral eccentricities, and tantrums, which then worried Jane. Jane began to detail Leslie's medical history. Every two weeks, if not more often, Leslie got sick with colds, which developed into wheezing, coughing, and labored breathing. Her constant absences from school caused her mother to miss work often.

Using an EAV (electro acupuncture) testing procedure, I found that Leslie was sensitive to milk, cheese, calcium, wheat, fruits, chocolate, sugars, salt, chloride, yeast, food additives, food coloring, modified starch, sulfites, toothpaste, beta-carotene, and vitamins A, B, and C. Besides foods, the list of her sensitivities included fabrics, dyes, down feathers, perfumes, mold, dust, pollen, flowers, grasses, chemicals, animals, fumes, and heat and cold. When I performed an enzyme evaluation, I found that she was unable to digest sugars and fats. I immediately prescribed an enzyme formula to help her digest sugars and fats. I also recommended protease enzymes to help fight infections in her body and strengthen her immune system. Then I began to clear her with BioSET for her many sensitivities.

Leslie responded immediately. She stopped getting sick as often, and her need for drugs diminished. After we had cleared her for sugars, her bouts with bronchitis and wheezing ceased almost entirely. Then I decided to visit her home to check which sensitivities she was encountering. I was not surprised to find that her bedroom was moldy, particularly an aquarium covered with algae. In fact, I was convinced from past experience that her lifelong asthma and wheezing were largely caused by her exposure to mold and mildew. After I cleared Leslie with BioSET for the specific mold found in her bedroom, her health changed dramatically. She has not missed a day of school in two years now, and she rarely experiences a runny nose or sore throat. Her coughing, wheezing, sleepless nights and, most importantly, her life-threatening breathing problems are gone.

Infectants: Bacteria, Viruses, and Parasites

The following case histories detail instances in which bacteria, viruses, and parasites were the triggers for symptoms.

Case 2: Jenny

Jenny, the two-year-old daughter of a family I was seeing for sensitivity clearings, experienced severe fevers, runny nose, and wheezing for no apparent reason. Her mother, Jodie, seemed to recall that these symptoms first occurred when her daughter was teething. She also commented that Jenny's breath was exceptionally foul when she was teething, which seemed unusual for a two-year-old.

Concerned that Jenny might have some bacteria in her mouth that were causing an occasional gum infection, I performed EAV testing and uncovered three specific bacteria sensitivities. Then I cleared Jenny with BioSET and recommended that she take protease for about ten days. I also suggested that Jodie clear her daughter at home if necessary for another week, to reinforce the clearing. Twenty-four hours later Jenny's fever was gone and she was her normal self again, with sweet breath and tons of energy. Since this clearing she has not experienced any problems with fever or wheezing.

Case 3: Hillary

A young woman named Hillary came to me for help with her chronic asthma, which had started when she was a child. She had been in and out of hospitals and on and off medications (including antibiotics) her whole life. When she coughed and wheezed, which she did often, she would bring up large quantities of colored mucus. I cleared her for many sensitivities, including pollen, flowers, dust, and many foods, and I recommended enzymes for protein digestion and sugar digestion, as well as protease three times a day to boost her immune system. These clearings improved her energy level and reduced the tightness in her chest and the frequency of her infections.

However, it was not until I cleared her for bacteria, viruses, fungi, and parasites that her asthma totally abated. It took quite a few clearings to clear the fungi, but fewer to clear the bacteria. Now Hillary no longer displays infectious symptoms such as excess or colored mucus and chronic coughing. Her need for her inhaler has decreased, and she is pleased that these improvements have maintained themselves so well. We have also cleared her environmental sensitivities.

Case 4: Michael

Michael, a two-year-old, had chronic coughing and ear infections every other month. His mother, Ester, commented that she could not remember a day when her son hadn't coughed. His breathing at night was labored, and he would scream with pain from ear infections. Impatient with the conventional medical program of constant antibiotics, cough medicine, and pain pills, Ester had tried homeopathy and some natural medicines without noticing any relief or change. She was another desperate mother who had come to me as a last resort.

With testing, I discovered that Michael was sensitive to all the ten basic sensitivities (amino acids, biochemicals, fatty acids, minerals, phenolics, sugars, vitamin A, B vitamins, vitamin C, and vitamin E) except iron as well as to wheat, yeast, some vegetables and fruits (especially avocado, oranges, carrots, string beans, bananas, apples, and pears), and to many bacteria and viruses. I began to clear Michael with BioSET for the basic sensitivities. He showed some improvement after being cleared for amino acids and vitamin C, which cleared his sensitivity to the vegetables and fruit. Then I cleared him for the B vitamins, which are an important precursor to the clearings for sugars, yeast, and grains. These clearings, in turn, can be the cornerstones of eliminating an asthmatic condition or any respiratory problem.

Michael was so sensitive to the B vitamins that he needed separate clearings for each one. Fortunately, his mother was able to do the clearings at home. When he came to the BioSET clinic for his next visit, he had completely cleared his sensitivity to B vitamins. Mom and Dad were feeling hopeful.

I then proceeded to complete the basic clearings. Although Michael was now only coughing occasionally on three out of seven nights, I was still not satisfied. I wanted him to be symptom-free. I decided to clear him for several environmental sensitivities, such as dust, mold, animals, pollen, and fabrics, and then for bacteria. During three different visits he was tested on all the bacteria and was cleared for the ones to which he was sensitive. In the many years since we have cleared these sensitivities, he has not had a single ear infection or cold. This case illustrates the axiom that nothing is normal except good health all the time. BioSET clearings for food and environmental sensitivities can help make this possible.

Poor Digestion: Sugar and Protein Intolerances

The following case history profiles a case where metabolism issues were the basis of asthmatic symptoms and clearly the key stressor dealt with during BioSET therapy.

Case 5: Sarah

Sarah, a fifty-four-year-old woman with a lifelong history of asthma and chronic sinusitis, had tried every therapy, including ones I had never heard of, to help control her asthma. For eight years she had experienced a series of sinus, ear, and respiratory infections that had required her to take a course of antibiotics every other month. She also told me that she suffered from acute food cravings, especially sugars, and that she always wanted to have something sweet in her mouth, although she managed to restrain herself most of the time. Much to her dismay, she was also unable to taste the foods she ate. She was severely underweight, chronically fatigued, and depressed about her condition. Sarah had been referred to me by someone at work whose food cravings, chronic colds, and flu had improved through the use of enzymes. She had decided to try yet another approach to see if it would help restore her health. Although she wasn't hopeful, she wasn't ready to give up either.

A thorough enzyme and nutritional evaluation revealed that Sarah was intolerant to sugars and protein. People who are intolerant to protein are unable to digest it, which can lead to a deficiency of amino acids and an inability to make the sugars that are needed to fuel the brain and energize the body. It was no wonder that Sarah craved sugars, and that every time she ate them they caused an accumulation of mucus. I immediately prescribed enzymes to support her digestion of sugars and protein, and I also recommended a protease enzyme as a natural boost to her immune system. Her recommended diet consisted of completely eliminating breads, fruits, and sugars of all kinds and minimizing her dairy intake. I recommended that she eat no more than one six-ounce serving of animal protein per day but unlimited servings of vegetable protein. Since starting this diet and enzyme regimen, Sarah has not had one episode of asthma and has no more chronic cough.

Food Coloring and Additives

Food coloring is another potential irritant that can bring on asthma attacks.

Case 6: Emily

Emily, a seventy-five-year-old woman, came to my office one day with labored breathing and wheezing. Since we had already cleared all the foods she was currently eating, she couldn't understand what had caused such a strong reaction. We had reviewed her diet at least three times, when suddenly she remembered that she had begun to cough right after someone had given her a butterscotch candy. When I cleared her for food coloring, her labored breathing ceased.

The message here is that we should never underestimate any potential food allergen. Even a taste of something you are sensitive to can cause asthma, a migraine, dizziness, eczema, or other chronic symptoms. BioSET practitioners see this phenomenon every day. As a matter of fact, some recent scientific research indicates that an individual can even react to the cooking steam of a sensitive food. Even the smell of fresh coffee brewing or the whiff of a certain spice can induce a reaction.

Case 7: Allan

A young patient named Allan, who had already been cleared with BioSET for some basic food sensitivities, including eggs, milk, and sugars, came to me complaining of wheezing and chest congestion. His mother wasn't sure what had brought on his asthma. When I asked what Allan had eaten the day before, he mentioned that he had ordered a salad at a salad-bar restaurant but had avoided the sugared dressings. I know from experience that such restaurants tend to use a variety of food additives and preservatives, such as hydrolyzed vegetable protein, MSG, sodium nitrate, nitrite, sulfur dioxide, BHT, and BHA, to preserve the foods in the salad bar and keep them fresh looking, which can trigger asthma.

When I tested Allan for food additives, he showed a significant reaction relative to the lung and respiratory meridians. Since I didn't know which additive was the culprit, however, I cleared him for all of them. Immediately after the clearing, his wheezing stopped. I suggested to his parents that if he started to wheeze at all during the next twenty-five hours, they should perform the BioSET procedure for fifteen minutes, to reinforce the clearing and prevent him from losing its effects. After being cleared for this sensitivity, Allan no longer had to avoid food additives.

Inhalants: Cleaners and Dust

Sensitivity clearings for dust and mold are extremely important for asthma sufferers. Although both are hardly visible, they can be life threatening, and most asthma patients need to be cleared for them.

Case 8: Gabrielle

Gabrielle, my daughter, always had difficulty breathing through her nose and was a mouth breather for the first two years of her life. She also had excess mucus in her throat that would cause occasional wheezing, sore throats, coughing, and an accumulation of fluid in her middle ear. I became concerned because this fluid accumulation seemed to be causing hearing difficulties. Gabrielle had been taking enzymes since infancy and had never had an infection or needed antibiotics. I took Gabrielle to a homeopathic pediatrician who experimented with many remedies, but none seemed to help her. Then I took her to a pediatric ear, eye, nose, and throat specialist who, after a five-minute examination, recommended having tubes put in her middle ear, along with a tonsillectomy and an adenoidectomy.

Although I listened with an open mind, I decided to seek one more opinion before signing her up for surgery. The pediatrician we consulted this time said, "Your daughter has allergies or sensitivities!" She also said that my daughter's hearing was not impaired, nor was she a candidate for surgery. Since I had just started using BioSET in my practice, I decided to clear Gabrielle myself. First, I cleared her for eggs and amino acids, which she craved—usually a sure indication that someone is sensitive to a particular food. Her craving stopped immediately. Then I cleared her for a mixture of vitamin C and strawberries, citrus, and some vegetables. Her mucus production diminished considerably, but she continued to snore. After I cleared her for the remaining ten basic sensitivities, she did not need to clear her throat anymore. Next, I cleared her for virus, yeast, and candida. Her hearing was now normal, and she no longer had fluid in her ear. But she still snored! What could the problem be? I was baffled.

Early one Sunday morning, Gabrielle and I were playing in her room. I opened the blinds and noticed dust flying around the room. I had not yet cleared her for dust, which I was sensitive to myself as a child. After cleaning her room thoroughly, I cleared her for dust with BioSET. That was fourteen years ago, and she has not snored, nor wheezed since.

Case 9: Aaron

At fifteen, my son, Aaron, was supposed to clean his own room and do his own laundry but, like a typical teenager, he would put it off for days, weeks, even longer. One night he woke up wheezing and complained that he couldn't breathe very well. Since he had spent the day in his room doing his homework, I figured there had to be something there that had triggered the attack. When I suggested it might be mattress dust, he confessed that he hadn't washed his sheets for some time—I didn't want to know how long! I stripped his bed, vacuumed his mattress, and dusted and cleaned his room, and he slept well that night. The next day, I cleared him with BioSET for the mattress dust I had saved from the vacuum cleaner. Since then, Aaron has never had any problems with wheezing or coughing. And I don't think he will ever put off washing his sheets again!

Inhalants: Chemicals and Animal Dander

The following case history describes instances of environmental stress, specifically involving chemicals or animal dander.

Case 10: Susan

Susan, a forty-one-year-old woman, came to see me with severe sensitivities that had caused eye tearing, fatigue, and asthma since childhood. In addition to being seasonal, her asthma attacks seemed to be triggered by foods and other environmental allergens. In particular, she suspected that chemical sensitivities were causing her eyes to tear. I did a complete workup, including sensitivity testing and an enzyme evaluation, and then cleared her for the basic substances she was sensitive to—amino acids, minerals, B vitamins, sugars, and salt. After being cleared for B vitamins, she felt a significant positive change in her health, and she has not had any asthma or labored breathing since.

Our next major accomplishment was clearing Susan's chronically reddened, teary eyes, which were not improved by the basic sensitivity clearings. After being cleared for some environmental sensitivities, such as perfumes, chemicals, hair products, and makeup (eye shadow, mascara, and blush), her eye symptoms almost entirely disappeared. However, it was not until the BioSET clearing for cat and other animal dander that these symptoms were completely eliminated.

Inhalants: Pollens, Perfume, and Smoke

The following case history involves various inhalants, including tobacco smoke, pollens, and even perfume!

Case 11: Sarah

Remember Sarah, whom I talked about earlier, the patient who had a complete reversal of her asthma symptoms with enzyme therapy and dietary changes, but still suffered chronic sinus congestion, an inability to taste foods, and some chronic eye irritation? When I tested her on environmental sensitivities, I found that she was still sensitive to grasses, trees, flowers, and pollens from a few different seasons. These types of sensitivities need to be cleared with BioSET *during* those seasons. She was also sensitive to perfume, cosmetics, tobacco smoke, and certain chemicals (including chlorine). After these specific clearings, her sinus congestion greatly diminished and her taste began to return, which was a dramatic and welcome change for her.

Inhalants: Wallpaper Fumes

The following case study describes an instance where the culprit was wallpaper fumes and other inhalants.

Case 12: Rachel

Rachel, a nineteen-year-old woman, had grown up with asthma and had used an inhaler for most of her life. Fortunately, she had never been hospitalized for a severe asthma attack, but she did notice her symptoms worsening as she got older. Overweight and fatigued most of the time, she had poor digestion and reported that she always had congestion in her lungs and woke up in the morning coughing as though she were a smoker, although she had never smoked. Every other month she seemed to come down with a cold, a flu, or bronchitis. Rachel had worked in many different environments, including a hair salon, a nightclub, and her mother's real estate business.

I immediately prescribed enzymes to help her breathing and enhance her immune response. Testing indicated that her poor digestion was due to an intolerance to fats. I encouraged her to eat a diet low in fat, which meant low in animal protein since meat tends to contain large amounts of fat. I prescribed enzymes to help digest fat and a good fatty-acid supplement. At the same time, I began to clear her with BioSET for all the basic sensitivities. Subsequent clearings included artificial sweeteners, dust, smog, exhaust, gas heat, radiation, paint, hair and nail chemicals, cosmetics, soaps, fabrics, formaldehyde, and carpets, as well as trees, flowers, and pollens. This was done over a two-month period.

Rachel improved in some ways, but she still experienced asthma attacks every night. We couldn't figure out what the trigger might be. Before I went to her house to check, I asked her, "Is there anything at all in your bedroom that you might have overlooked?" She went home and checked every inch of her room to find out what could possibly be triggering her asthma. When she returned to my office, she was carrying a piece of grass cloth wallpaper, which was the only thing for which we had not tested. As it turned out, she was definitely sensitive to her wallpaper and even felt her chest tighten up when she held it. After I cleared her for the wallpaper using BioSET, she noticed immediate results, including instantaneous relief in her chest. It has been ten years since this clearing, and she has been well ever since.

Inhalant: Smoke

This next story reveals the stress that smoking can put on the health of a sensitive individual.

Case 13: Susan

After being symptom-free for three years, Susan recently came to see me with red and irritated eyes. She thought perhaps she was reacting to some new makeup she had begun to use. Using BioSET testing procedures, we discovered that she was sensitive to tobacco smoke and solar radiation, causing stress in her spleen and kidney meridians.

At first Susan couldn't remember coming into contact with smoke, and she avoided exposing herself to the sun. As we talked, however, she recalled that she had been staying with someone who was a smoker and had actually smoked a few cigarettes herself. When she was tested three years before, she had been extremely sensitive to smoke of all kinds, so it wasn't a surprise to see her react so dramatically now. What was surprising was that she had not had an asthmatic attack since our last visit, despite the exposure to smoke.

Susan was cleared for smoke that day, and she has been fine ever since.

Vitamin Deficiency and Antioxidants

The next case history delves into vitamin and other metabolic deficiencies.

Case 14: Carey

Carey, a thirty-two-year-old woman, came to see me complaining of chronic sinus infection, postnasal drip, and a recurring cough. She was aware that some allergens (perfumes, chemicals, formaldehyde, and certain foods) made her health worse. After an extensive workup, I found that she tested positive to all the basic sensitivities, with the most severe being vitamin C and the bioflavonoids. An enzyme and detoxification evaluation revealed liver and bowel toxicity. When I started her on some enzymes for digestion and for liver detoxification and repair, I simultaneously began to clear her with BioSET for her basic sensitivities.

After clearing her for vitamin C and supplementing her diet with a vitamin C and antioxidants enzyme (including pau d'arco, garlic, and grape seed extract), Carey experienced dramatic positive changes in her health, including freedom from sinus congestion and coughing. Antioxidants are essential tools for the detoxification of free radicals, which, if not detoxified, can result in severe damage to body tissues. She also remarked that her lifelong food cravings had diminished. Her energy had significantly increased, and she was all smiles each time I saw her in the following weeks.

Evidence has shown that patients should always supplement their diet with a vitamin or mineral after desensitization to that nutrient because they are usually deficient in the substance due to their former inability to utilize it. Symptoms can change rather quickly when supplementation takes place. Some vitamins need long-term supplementation, others only short-term. Each person is different, and there are several testing procedures to evaluate the need for supplementation.

Enzyme Deficiencies

This case study examines the implications of enzymes in health problems.

Case 15: Betty

Years ago, before I started to practice BioSET, Betty came to see me with symptoms of heartburn, severe bloating, swelling of her abdomen, and an inability to digest anything she ate. She also noted that over the last two years, she had suffered from a chronic cough and periods of shortness of breath. At sixty-six, she was slim and healthy in every other way and did not take any medication, which is unusual for a woman her age. In addition, her diet was impeccably well balanced, and she watched her intake of fat and sugar. Her complexion and her coloring were excellent. She walked a mile every day and did yoga two to three times per week.

When I performed a complete enzyme evaluation and a thorough investigation of her diet, I found a significant amount of gastric distress. Betty had reported that she experienced reflux and nausea after eating many days of the week. After prescribing a gastric enzyme to help neutralize her acidic stomach, I spent time with her reviewing her diet. Although she consumed no coffee, it turned out that she adored chocolate and could not let a day go by without having some. She also mentioned that, following a friend's recommendation, she had increased her calcium intake through both calcium supplements and dairy products to avoid the onset of osteoporosis. As a child, Betty remembered having trouble digesting milk but thought she had outgrown it.

Further examination indicated that she was suffering from reflux and gastritis. Sure enough, the foods she was eating that were high in oxalic acid, such as chocolate, dairy, and calcium, seemed to be contributing to her digestive problems. Since these problems could worsen over time, I advised her to ease off the chocolate, temporarily eliminate her calcium intake, and avoid foods high in oxalic acid.

The combination of a dietary modification and supplementary enzymes prompted her to call me two weeks later to say that her coughing was almost completely gone and she had not felt this good in years. I reminded her that she could also take her enzymes after meals, as needed, to eliminate the coughing, which she did with success.

Foods: Chocolate

The following case history examines the implications of food sensitivities, specifically chocolate.

Case 16: Betty

Three years later Betty came to see me again, after hearing that I was now using a unique desensitization technique called BioSET. She remembered my comment that she was possibly sensitive to calcium and oxalates and wondered if she might also be sensitive to chocolate. She hadn't been able to eliminate it from her diet for long and continued to crave it. She noted that her bloating had returned but that her coughing and shortness of breath were completely gone and had never returned. Betty was still concerned about calcium deficiency and its long-term effects, such as arthritis, osteoporosis, insomnia, and nervousness. She had recently begun to experience cramping and some shaking in her legs, which could have been the result of a calcium deficiency.

I began by testing her on an expanded group of basic sensitivities. As I suspected, I found her sensitive to calcium, sugars, vitamin C, chocolate, and other vitamins. After repeating a thorough enzyme evaluation, I found that she had gastric reflux, just as before. She admitted that she had taken her enzymes for one year and then had discontinued them because she was feeling better. However, she had kept to her gastritis diet, except for the chocolate, her mad love.

This time I cleared her with BioSET over the course of a few weeks for dairy (including milk and yogurt), sugars, phenolics, and a few other sensitivities. She resumed her calcium supplements with no deleterious effect and began eating dairy products again with no bloating. She was also able to end her love affair with chocolate for the first time in her life. "Dr. Ellen," she said, "this is the first time I can walk past a See's Candy store and resist the urge to have some chocolate." She noticed immediately that she was sleeping better, her legs had stopped shaking, and the joint pain she had been experiencing lessened. Good protein digestion helps with the absorption of calcium.

Foods: Sugars

The next case study examines the role of sugar sensitivity and digestion in health problems.

Case 17: Jonathan

Jonathan is a healthy young man who grew up on good nutrition and enzymes for proper digestion. He has never been on a prescription antibiotic because he was always prescribed enzymes. When he was two years old, his pediatrician, for no apparent reason, said his breathing sounded like an asthmatic's. His parents were alarmed and found it hard to believe, as neither of them had ever been diagnosed with asthma. Since Jonathan had a slight cold at the time, they decided to disregard the pediatrician's comment and never really thought about it again.

The year Jonathan turned fourteen, he developed a chronic cough that commenced in January and lasted until his birthday in the beginning of March. The cough recurred each year when the weather was damp.

One evening Jonathan's mother was talking on the phone with her ninety-five-year-old grandmother, who overheard her grandson coughing and said, "Becky, you used to have the same cough when you were fourteen years old." This made Becky wonder whether she would have been diagnosed as an asthmatic if physicians back then had been as quick to diagnose asthma as they are today. She had, however, been diagnosed with allergies and began allergy shots. This memory was significant for Becky, since she knew that hereditary factors play a key role in children's sensitivities, though she had never made the connection between her childhood sensitivities and her children's.

The discovery of her son's allergies and sensitivities led her to the BioSET clinic, where he was tested and cleared for his basic sensitivities. One interesting observation that emerged was that Jonathan coughed whenever he ate sugar, something he rarely did. He did love natural sodas, however, which contain large quantities of high fructose corn syrup. This sweetener is high in sugar and can often be a trigger for asthmatics. After he was cleared for sugars, Jonathan's coughing and wheezing completely disappeared.

Foods: Wheat

The following case study deals with the far-reaching implications of a wheat sensitivity.

Case 18: Eric

A little boy named Eric, who was not quite two, was brought to the BioSET clinic with a chronic cough and regular, labored breathing. His mother, who traveled often for her work, had become afraid to leave him because of the special care and attention he needed. She was also concerned that the antibiotics and steroids he was regularly prescribed were actually making him more susceptible to ear and upper respiratory infections. In my clinic, I have seen people of all ages negatively affected by corticosteroids, which inhibit the immune system.

Eric was tested and cleared with BioSET for the basic food sensitivities. Calcium and soy proved to be an extremely important clearing for him because his mother had him on soy formula, which is high in calcium. Since the sugar clearing, Eric has not had one ear infection or any need for antibiotics.

However, the most dramatic allergens in relationship to his coughing and labored breathing were salt and wheat. Many asthmatic attacks are triggered by salt, a substance that occurs naturally in many foods, such as celery, cucumbers, citrus, and water. Wheat is another key sensitivity for asthmatics, and clearing for it was a turning point for Eric. Even though a clearing for wheat helps reduce cravings for that food, I recommend that clients rarely eat wheat due to its damaging effects on health. Once Eric was cleared for wheat with BioSET, and consequently reduced his intake of that food, his coughing, congestion, and labored breathing were eliminated. He is now able to eat small amounts of wheat, soy, and dairy products without any problems.

Environment: Sick Building

The following case history reveals the stress that the environments of certain buildings can have on their inhabitants.

Case 19: Lisa

Lisa, a woman in her forties, suffered so severely from eczema, breathing difficulties, and sinus congestion that her many physicians had lost hope of restoring her to health. I proceeded to try to clear some of her symptoms with BioSET. She was prescribed a multiple enzyme formula to help her digest protein and carbohydrates, as well as an enzyme formula high in amylase to help reduce inflammation. After a few weeks, I recommended a liver-detoxifying enzyme, antioxidants, and bowel cleansers.

When a month later Lisa still showed no improvement, I did some detective work. She told me that she had noticed a dramatic worsening of her symptoms after she had begun working in her current office building. Many of her fellow employees, she said, were chronically sick with flu, sore throats, and breathing problems, and she wondered about the safety of her working environment, which was located on a floor without any windows.

During the energy crisis, I explained to her, we began to insulate and seal our buildings more thoroughly. This saved energy, but caused pollutants to be trapped indoors, possibly creating havoc in the human body. After some thought, I decided to clear Lisa first for chemicals and then for the air in her office, which she collected in a jar left open in the office overnight. After the first clearing her eczema improved dramatically, and after the second her breathing cleared up completely.

Contactants: Feathers

The following case history descirbes one patient's common contactant sensitivity to feathers.

Case 20: Kelly

A woman in her late twenties named Kelly came to the BioSET clinic for chronic sinusitis, a chronic cough, constant fatigue, and occasional asthma. She was overweight, and had seen me several years before for chiropractic for her lower back. Recently, she had heard that I was clearing food and environmental sensitivities and hoped that I could help her.

Testing indicated that she was sensitive to phenolics, B vitamins, sugars, minerals, and down feathers, and we cleared her for these basic sensitivities. It was especially important to clear feathers since Kelly slept with a down pillow, used a down comforter, and owned a down couch. The day after her clearing for feathers, she came in to see me to make sure she had been completely cleared. When she tested strong for the sensitivity (meaning there was no longer a reaction), she hugged and kissed me, explaining that this was the first morning she could remember having awakened without a runny nose and congestion. She was ecstatic that it would not be the last.

I then cleared her for her other sensitivities. After clearing her for yeast and candida, her fatigue diminished and her craving for bread disappeared. She began to lose weight after the clearings for yeast, wheat, and dairy.

Since that first clearing, Kelly has not had a problem with her sinuses, and her asthma and coughing are nonexistent. How many people do you know who use down blankets and pillows? Many are probably sensitive to them and wake up coughing and sneezing. Asthma sufferers should not use down accessories or pillows until they have been cleared for feathers with BioSET. This can certainly be done at home.

Hormones: Thyroid

The following case study examines one patient's sensitivities to hormones. People can be sensitive to hormones taken as supplements, as well as hormones secreted in their own bodies.

Case 21: Candace

One of the patients who came to the BioSET clinic, a sixty-seven-year-old woman named Candace who suffered from chronic emphysema and asthma, had tried everything for her breathing difficulties, which she had been experiencing for years. She lived a very healthy life otherwise. She ate a balanced diet of all organic foods, never used any alcohol, and had never smoked. However, her mother had died of emphysema, and she was frightened that she might be destined for the same fate.

Candace had been cleared with BioSET for many sensitivities, including foods, environmental sensitivities, drugs, and metabolic imbalances, which had helped curtail her bouts of coughing. But nothing seemed to have any effect on her breathing problems and her lung capacity. Understandably, these symptoms frightened her the most. One day she was cleared for her own thyroid hormones. The response was remarkable. Almost immediately her lung capacity expanded significantly, and the change has been long lasting.

The Ten Basic Sensitivities

This case history shows how BioSET deals with the most common sensitivities in the system.

Case 22: Michael

Michael, a thirty-one-year-old music producer, was referred by one of my patients. He had suffered from severe asthma since birth and could not go anywhere without his inhaler and drugs. He came to me hoping that he might be able to go off his medication. He was already aware that he was sensitive to house dust, cats, dogs, feathers, cigarette smoke, perfume, pollens, grasses, and certain climatic changes that aggravated his asthma.

I explained to him that I needed to test and clear him for the basic sensitivities before clearing him for some of the more obvious ones. Sure enough, he proved to be sensitive to all ten of the basic sensitivities.

Then I performed an in-depth nutritional analysis consisting of an enzyme assessment. I found him to be highly intolerant of proteins and sugars and unable to absorb certain nutrients. These intolerances may have caused not only his respiratory problems, but also his hypoglycemia, bloating, low adrenal function, fatigue, attention deficit problems, and low energy level. He began to take some enzymes to support his digestion of proteins and sugars. At the same time, I began clearing him with BioSET for the sensitivity groups.

After two months on the road, Michael called to tell me he had not had another asthma attack or used his medication since the clearing for the first group—the largest time span between attacks since he was six years old. After I finally finished clearing him for the ten basic sensitivities, I retested him for his known sensitivities, such as cats, dogs, pollens, and house dust, and found that he was no longer sensitive to any of them. When I spoke to Michael recently, he couldn't remember the last time he had coughed, let alone wheezed or used his inhaler. He said he is truly a different person.

Conclusion

In the United States, more than one out of every ten children between five and seventeen years old, approximately 6.2 million individuals, suffer from asthma. According to the American Lung Association, asthma attack–prevalence rates are highest in the five- to seventeen-year-old range.[1] Many of these children do not have control over their disease, although most parents would answer differently. Doctors are encouraging parents and caregivers to be more proactive and to unite to gain control over and conquer asthma.

BioSET is a system that is based on traditional and contemporary healing modalities and has been proven, via thousands of asthma success stories over the course of a decade, to be able to alleviate symptoms of sensitivities and asthma in anyone, from young children to the elderly. BioSET is not meant to be a substitute for a patient's present conventional treatment nor the ultimate cure for asthma, but is meant to complement and enhance other approaches in ameliorating an asthmatic's hypersensitive reactions and improving their digestion and absorption of foods, thereby decreasing the severity and frequency of asthma symptoms. If a patient is under the care of a BioSET practitioner, then BioSET can become the primary treatment. But even if a patient is under the care of another physician, BioSET can be a helpful adjunct to the current medication and conventional treatment.

I will never forget an experience I had while attending the American Bookseller Association sales conference in Chicago. While I was walking down the aisles at the show, holding my book in my arms, a woman enthusiastically tapped me on the shoulder. She said, "You don't know me, but I know you. I bought your *Food Allergy Cure* a year ago and began working with your system at home. I ordered the suggested enzymes and detoxification drops based on the self-evaluation questionnaire from your book, and began clearing my two sons, who have asthma, for the sensitivities suggested in your book. A year later, they both are 75 percent better, with very few asthma symptoms, infrequent use of their medication, and no missed school days. Last year because of asthma, they missed an average of fourteen days from school—way too much. I had to stop you and shake your hand and thank you for BioSET."

Recently, in June 2006, I was reading a news article on asthma. My heart ached when I read the story of a ten-year-old boy from Charlotte, North Carolina. This boy has not been able to play football with his friends for a very long time. He was being treated with cortisone injections, drug IVs, and more asthma medications every year, yet he was continually getting sick. For example, every time he came down with a cold, the next day he was taken to the hospital to receive emergency treatment for his asthma. This young boy is coping with his asthma due to his family's vigilant efforts to adhere to his prescribed treatment regimen. But I can't help but wonder what his results would be if he underwent BioSET sensitivity diagnosis and clearings in conjunction with his regular treatments.

BioSET is a holistic system based upon improving your lifestyle through a healthier diet, good digestion, detoxification, cleaning up your environment, and introducing green products that reduce sensitivity reactions. In addition, it minimizes your reactions to food and environmental sensitivities through clearings and desensitization of various items that impact your immune health and vitality.

Here's a different and very compelling scenario from the one above, which happened to another child. This one came to the BioSET clinic for evaluation a few weeks ago.

Samantha, aged seven, had suffered from asthma ever since she was three years old. She was in and out of the hospital emergency room often and was really not doing very well with her array of asthma medications. Her family was very diligent about monitoring her medications and caring for her, but their frustration mounted each year as Samantha's missed school days and swim practices continued to increase.

The family of one of Samantha's classmates referred her parents to our clinic. We assessed her digestion and toxicity status as well as her food and environmental sensitivities. We discovered that she was very sensitive to eggs, dairy, wheat, rice, chocolate, turkey, pork, some vegetables and fruits, her cat, dust, and grass pollen. She was also very sensitive to her cereal and the multivitamin she took daily. Samantha was taking medication every day for her sensitivities and asthma, and she used an inhaler three to four days a week to help control her episodes of wheezing and difficult breathing. Just like the boy discussed above, her worst times were when she came down with a cold. A simple cold would usually end up as bronchitis and/or a trip to the emergency room for more concentrated respiratory therapy.

We designed a BioSET protocol for Samantha, consisting of digestive enzymes, detoxification drops, dietary changes, and clearings for all of her sensitivities. Her mother also did some home clearings for water, pollen, and household air.

The results were outstanding. Soon thereafter, Samantha no longer needed any auxiliary medications, just her maintenance dose once a day. Not only does she rarely get any colds or infections, she has not needed to visit the emergency room since. Her mother said that she is a totally different girl—her asthma is controlled, her health is excellent, and her disposition has improved since she is able to avoid the stress of taking so many medications and living with the anxiety of not knowing what was going to happen to her from day to day.

Live Free from Asthma and Allergies is not for only a few individuals who suffer from extreme asthma, but for everyone who has ever been diagnosed with this disease. BioSET is a treatment option that is not harmful, dangerous, or expensive and is completely noninvasive. Its philosophy recognizes the great healing potential inside each of us, and the program assists our bodies in achieving our highest level of strength and well-being. If you think you can benefit from BioSET and wish to learn more, visit my website at www.bioset.net. Learning the art of prevention is the true essence of all natural health systems, and BioSET is no exception.

Appendices

Foods Related to Dietary Stress and Foods and Materials Containing Key Allergens

The research on allergies is extensive. Currently the Medline database of the National Library of Medicine, National Institutes of Health (NIH), contains hundreds of thousands of entries on allergies. Terms used to classify the research on allergies include the following:

+ Allergy: "Hypersensitivity caused by exposure to a particular allergen (antigen) resulting in a marked increase in reactivity . . . upon subsequent exposure sometimes resulting in harmful immunologic consequences."[1] (Medline includes 165,144 abstract summaries under the general term "allergy.")

+ Hypersensitivity: "Altered reactivity to an antigen, which can result in pathologic reactions upon subsequent exposure to that particular antigen."[2]

+ Hypersensitivity, Delayed: "An increased reactivity to specific antigens mediated not by antibodies but by cells."[3] (There are 19,714 Medline entries under hypersensitivity.)

+ Hypersensitivity, Immediate: "Hypersensitivity reactions which occur within minutes of exposure to a challenging antigen due to the release of histamine which follows the antigen-antibody reaction and causes smooth muscle contraction and increased vascular permeability."[4] (There are 7,159 of these Medline entries.)

+ Sensitivity: "An abnormal response to an allergen, drug or other external stimulus of the senses."[5]

The following lists reveal ingredients in foods that are common sensitivities for asthmatics.

Foods and Materials Containing Corn

Adhesives

Ale

American brandies: apple, grape

Aspirin and other tablets

Bacon

Baking mixes: Aunt Jemima Pancake Mix, Bisquick, Complete Pancake Mix, Doughnuts

Baking powders

Batters for frying meat, fish, fowl

Beers

Beets, Harvard

Beverages, carbonated

Bleached white flours

Bourbon and other whiskies

Breads and pastries

Cakes

Candy: box candies, candy bars, commercial candies

Catsups

Cheerios

Cheeses

Chili

Chop suey

Coffee, instant

Confectioner's sugar

Cookies

Corn: flakes, flour, meal, oil, parched, popped, starch, sugars (cerelose, dextrose, dyno), unripe (canned, fresh, fritters, frozen, roasting ears, succotash)

Cough syrups

Cream pies

Cream puffs

Cups, paper

Dates, confection

Deep fat frying mixtures

Dentifrices

Excipients or diluents in: capsules, suppositories, tablets, vitamins

Flour, bleached

Foods, fried

French dressing

Fritos

Frostings

Fruits

Frying fats

Gelatin capsules

Gelatin dessert

Gin

Glucose products

Graham crackers

Grape juice

Gravies

Grits

Gum on envelopes, stickers, stamps, tapes, labels

Gums, chewing

Ham, cured or tenderized

Hominy

Ice creams

Ices

Inhalants: bath powders, body powders, cooking fumes from fresh corn

Jams

Jellies

Jell-O

Kremel

Leavening agents: baking powders, yeasts

Liquors: ale, beer, gin, whiskey

Lozenges

Margarine

Milk in paper cartons

Monosodium glutamate

Nescafe

Ointments

Peanut butters

Peas, canned

Plastic food wrappers (the inner surfaces may be coated with cornstarch)

Powdered sugar

Preserves

Puddings: blanc mange, custards, Royal pudding

Rice, coated

Salad dressings

Salt: salt cellars in restaurants

Sandwich spreads

Sauces: sundaes, meats, fish, vegetables

Seasoned salt

Sherbets

Similac

String beans: canned, frozen

Soups: creamed, thickened, vegetable

Soybean milks

Starch

Starch fumes while ironing clothes

Syrups, commercially prepared: glucose, Karo

Talcums

Teas, instant

Toothpaste (some)

Tortillas

Vanillin

Vegetables: canned, creamed, frozen

Vinegar, distilled

Vitamins

Whiskies: bourbon, scotch

Wines, American*: dessert, fortified, sparkling

*Some brands are corn-free

Foods Containing Eggs

Baking powder

Batters for french frying

Bavarian cream

Boiled dressings

Bouillon

Bread

Breaded foods

Cake flour

Cakes

French toast

Fritters

Frosting

Glazed rolls

Griddle cakes

Hamburger mix

Hollandaise sauce

Ice cream

Ices

Icings

Macaroni

Macaroons

Malted cocoa drinks

Marshmallows

Meat jellies

Meat loaf

Meat patties

Meringues

Noodles

Ovaltine

Pancake flour

Pancakes

Pretzels

Pudding

Salad dressing

Sauces

Sausages

Sherbets

Souffles

Soups

Spaghetti

Spanish creams

Tartar sauce

Waffle mixes

Waffles

Wines

Foods Containing Milk

Baker's bread

Baking powder biscuits

Bavarian cream

Bisques

Blanc mange

Boiled salad dressings

Butter

Buttermilk

Butter sauces

Cakes

Candies

Cheeses

Chocolate

Chowders

Cocoa drinks, mixtures

Cookies

Cream

Creamed foods

Cream sauces

Curds

Custards

Doughnuts

Eggs, scrambled

Flour mixtures

Foods fried in butter (fish, poultry, beef, pork)

Foods prepared au gratin

Fritters

Gravies

Hamburgers

Hard sauces

Hash

Hotcakes

Ice creams

Malted milk

Margarine

Mashed potatoes

Meat loaf

Milk chocolate

Omelets

Ovaltine

Pie crust (some)

Prepared mixes: biscuits, cakes, cookies, doughnuts, muffins, pancakes, pie crust, waffles

Salad dressings

Sausages, cooked

Scalloped dishes

Sherbets

Soda crackers

Souffles

Soups

Whey

Foods and Materials Containing Formaldehyde

Formaldehyde is a formic aldehyde, a powerful disinfectant gas produced by the oxidation of methyl alcohol.* The aqueous solution is a colorless, volatile fluid used as a surgical and general antiseptic as well as a preservative. It is also utilized as a reagent, a substance used in detecting or analyzing another substance by chemical, microscopic, or other means.

Formaldehyde is commonly used in the following ways:

1. As an intermediate in the synthesis of alcohols, acids, and chemicals

2. In formulating slow-release nitrogen fertilizers and in destroying microorganisms responsible for plant disease

3. As a tanning agent

4. As a rodent poison

5. As an added agent to make concrete, plaster, and related products impermeable to liquids

6. In antiperspirants and antiseptics in dentrifices, mouthwashes, and germicidal and detergent soaps

7. In hair setting lotions and shampoos

8. As an air deodorant in public places and in industrial environments

9. In destroying bacteria, fungi, molds, and yeasts

10. In disinfecting equipment in the fermentation industry and the manufacture of antibiotics

11. In disinfecting sickrooms and surgical instruments

12. In the synthesis of dyes, stripping agents, and various specialty chemicals in the dye industry

13. In the manufacture of embalming fluids when combined with alcohol, glycerol, and phenol

14. In preserving products such as waxes, polishes, adhesives, fats, oils, and anatomical specimens

15. In the synthesis of explosives

16. In preparing fireproofing compositions to apply to fabrics in conjunction with other chemicals

17. In insecticidal solutions for killing flies, mosquitoes, and moths

18. In the synthesis of vitamin A and to improve the activity of vitamin E preparations

19. In improving set strength and water resistance in paper products

20. In preserving and accelerating photographic developing solutions

21. In making natural and synthetic fibers crease resistant, wrinkle resistant, crushproof, water repellent, dye-fast, flame resistant, water resistant, shrinkproof, mothproof (wool), and more elastic (wood)

22. In making synthetic resins, wood veneer (for wallpaper), and artificial aging, and reduction of shrinkage in wood preservation

23. As part of wallboard in construction of houses and apartments

24. As a resin in nail polish and an undercoating of nail polish

* Formaldehyde accounts for about 50 percent of the estimated total aldehydes in polluted air. The major sources of aldehyde pollution are in the incomplete combustions of hydrocarbons in gasoline and diesel engines, the burning of fuels, and incineration waste. Formaldehyde is believed to be the principal agent responsible for burning the eyes in smog. Aldehydes can also react further to form additional products such as ozone.

Foods and Materials Containing Hydrocarbons

Hydrocarbons are organic compounds comprised of hydrogen and carbon. If the geological concept that conifer forests are the precursors of the original sources of the hydrocarbons—coal, oil, gas—is valid, then we should consider these materials as well. Such an interpretation is indicated by the similar clinical effects of pine and its combustion products with those of coal, oil, and gas and their combustion products and derivatives.

Hydrocarbons are commonly used in the following products:

1. Alcohol

2. Artificially colored foods and drugs

3. Burning green wood, which contains considerable oil and resin

4. Cements and other adhesives

5. Cleaning fluids and lighter fluids

6. Creosote-impregnated wood

7. Oil evaporating from mechanical devices

8. Evaporative paints, varnish, and other solvents

9. Foods exposed to gas for ripening, roasting, or clarifying through bone char that is reactivated in gas-fired ovens

10. Fuel, including coal, oil, gas, diesel and nondiesel, and their combustion

11. Garage odors, which foul the air of living quarters

12. Industrial and agricultural chemicals, which contaminate water supplies

13. Insecticides

14. Mineral oil

15. Miscellaneous odors, including detergents, soaps containing naphtha, ammonia, bleach, cleansing powders containing bleach, window-washing compounds, certain silver- and brass-polishing materials, and deodorants and disinfectants (especially pine-scented)

16. Newsprint

17. Oil-soluble food sprays that permeate the cooking surface to which they are applied and cannot be removed by washing, peeling, soaking in water or vinegar, or by cooking

18. Paraffins used in coating and scaling, in candles, in rubber compounding, in pharmaceuticals, and in cosmetics

19. Pine oil exposure

20. Plastics produced by chemical condensations

21. Refrigerants (Freon) and spray containers

22. Roofing and road construction compounds

23. Sponge rubber

Foods and Materials Containing Soybeans

Automobile parts: Some automobile manufacturers are using soybeans to make a plastic that is used to make window frames, steering wheels, gearshift knobs, distributors, and other parts. They also make an upholstery fabric from soybeans.

Bakery goods: Many bakers now use soybean flour containing only 1 percent oil in their dough mixtures for breads, cakes, rolls, and pastries. This keeps baked goods moist and salable several days longer. Toasted soybeans are used in place of peanuts on breakfast rolls. Biscuits and several crisp crackers have soybean flour in them.

Candies: Soy flours are used in hard candies, fudge, nut candies, custards, and caramels. Lecithin is invariably derived from soybeans for use in candies, particularly chocolate, to prevent drying out and to emulsify the fats.

Industrial and other contactants: Soy products are used in varnish, paints, enamels, printing ink, massage creams, candles, celluloid, linoleum, adhesives, paper finishes, blankets, cloth, nitroglycerine, urease, pet food, soaps, fertilizers, and automobile parts. It is also used for fodder, textile dressing, glycerine, and coffee substitutes and to make lubricating and illuminating oil. Soybeans are used to make rubber substitutes, and its lecithin is used as a stabilizer in leaded gasoline.

Meats: Pork link sausage and lunch meats can contain soybeans. The allergic individual should buy only pure meat products.

Milk substitutes: Some bakeries use soymilk instead of cow's milk in recipes.

Miscellaneous: Soy products are used in some ice creams and in many soups. Fresh green soy sprouts are served as a vegetable, especially in Chinese dishes. Soybeans are roasted, salted, and used in place of peanuts. They are used to make soy noodles, macaroons, and spaghetti. Some seasonings contain soy, as do a number of frying fats and shortenings. Oleomargarines and butter substitutes contain the oil and bean products. It is also present in many cookies, crackers, and snacks.

Salad dressings and sauces: Many salad dressings and mayonnaises contain soy oil but only show on the label that they contain vegetable oil. When using a particular brand of dressing or mayonnaise, inquire as to the contents.

Note: Keep in mind that soybeans and their products are used as flour, oil, and milk, and soybean nuts are commonly served. We are living in an era of expanding uses for soybeans, and the allergy sufferer should anticipate many possible contacts. Additionally, as new food combinations become popular, many new contacts can be expected. When undergoing a BioSET treatment for soybeans, eat only foods in their original form. Avoid baked, processed, and packaged foods. Wear cotton or leather gloves and a mask when handling or coming in close proximity (less than four feet) with the products on the above list.

Foods Containing Hidden Sugars

BEVERAGES

Cola drinks

Cordials

Ginger ale

Orangeade

Root beer

7UP soft drink

Soda pop

Sweet cider

Whiskey sour

CAKES AND COOKIES

Angel food

Applesauce cake

Brownies (plain)

Cheesecake

Chocolate cake

Chocolate cookies

Chocolate éclair

Coffee cake

Cream puff

Cupcake (iced)

Doughnuts (glazed)

Doughnuts (plain)

Fig Newtons cookies

Fruitcake

Gingersnaps

Jelly roll

Macaroons

Nut cookies

Oatmeal cookies

Orange cake

Pound cake

Sponge cake

Strawberry shortcake

Sugar cookies

CANDIES

Chewing gum
Chocolate (cream filling)
Chocolate mints
Fudge

Hard candy
Hershey's candy bar
Life Savers candy
Peanut brittle

CANNED FRUITS AND JUICES

Apricots
Apricot syrup
Fruit cocktail
Fruit juice (sweetened)

Fruit syrup
Peaches
Stewed fruits

DAIRY PRODUCTS

Ice cream
Ice cream bar
Ice cream cone

Ice cream soda
Ice cream sundae
Milk shake

JAMS, JELLIES, AND DESSERTS

Apple butter
Apple cobbler
Custard
French pastry

Jell-O
Jelly
Orange marmalade

Foods Containing Wheat

BEVERAGES

Beer

Cocomalt

Gin (any drink with grain-
neutral spirits)

Malted milk

Ovaltine

Postum

Whiskey

BREADS

Biscuits

Breads: corn, gluten, graham,
rye, soy, wheat

Crackers

Muffins

Popovers

Pretzels

Rolls

CEREALS

All wheat cereals

Bran flakes

Corn flakes

Cream of wheat

Grapenuts

Other malted cereals

Puffed wheat

Rice Krispies

Shredded wheat

Triscuits

FLOURS

Buckwheat

Corn

Gluten

Graham

Lima bean

Rye

White

Whole wheat

PASTRIES AND DESSERTS

Cakes
Candy bars
Chocolate candy
Cookies

Doughnuts
Frozen pies
Pies
Puddings

WHEAT PRODUCTS

Bread
Dumplings
Macaroni
Noodles

Rusk
Spaghetti
Vermicelli
Zweiback

MISCELLANEOUS

Bouillon cubes
Chocolate candy
Chocolate (except bitter cocoa and bitter chocolate)
Cooked mixed meat dishes
Fats that have been used for frying
Foods rolled in flour
Gravies
Griddle cakes
Hotcakes
Ice cream cones
Matzos

Mayonnaise
Most cooked and prepared meat: sausages, hot dogs, bologna, liverwurst, luncheon ham, hamburger
Pancake mixes
Sauces
Some yeasts
Synthetic pepper
Thickening in ice cream
Waffles
Wheat cakes
Wheat germ

Foods Containing Yeast

The following foods contain yeast as an additive ingredient during preparation (often called leavening):

Breads

Cake and cake mixes

Canned icebox biscuits

Cookies

Crackers

Hamburger buns

Hot dog buns

Meat fried in cracker crumbs

Milk fortified with vitamins from yeast

Pastries

Pretzels

Rolls, homemade or canned

The following substances contain yeast or yeast-like substances because of their nature or the nature of their manufacture or preparation:

Buttermilk

Cheeses of all kinds, including cottage cheese

Citrus fruit juices, frozen or canned (only home-squeezed are yeast free!)

Fermented beverages, including whiskey, wine, brandy, gin, rum, vodka, and root beer

Malted products, including cereals, candy, and malted milk drinks

Mushrooms

Truffles

Vinegars (apple, pear, grape, and distilled). These may be used alone or in such foods as catsup, mayonnaise, olives, pickles, sauerkraut, condiments, horseradish, French dressing, salad dressing, barbecue sauce, tomato sauce, chili peppers, mince pie, and Gerber's Oatmeal and Barley Cereal

The following products contain substances that are derived from yeast or have their source in yeast. *Read all labels!*

Capsules or tablets containing vitamin B made from yeast

Multiple vitamins

Some enzyme supplements containing brewer's yeast

Vitamin B capsules or tablets made from yeast

Drugs Containing No Corn, Wheat, or Milk

Accutane Capsules

Acetaminophen

Allerest Children's Chewable Tablets

Allerest Eye Drops

Allerest Nasal Spray

Amphojel Suspension

Amphojel Suspension without Flavor

Anaprox

Ancef Injection

Aspirin Uniserts

Bacitracin Sterile

Bacitracin Suspension

Bacitracin Tablets

Bacitracin Topical Ointment

Basaljel Suspension

Basaljel Suspension Extra Strength

Benedryl Steri-Vial

Berocca Plus Tablets

Berocca Tablets

Bisacodyl (Dulcolax)

Brexin L.A. Capsules

Cafergot Suppositories

Calciferol Drops

Castor oil

Casufru liquid

Cedilanid-D Injection

Cerose compound capsules

Cerubidine Injectable

Chardose powder

Chloromycetin Cream 1 Percent

Chloromycetin Opthalmic Ointment

Chloromycetin Palmitate Oral Suspension

Chloromycetin Sodium Succinate Steri-Vial

Chromagen capsules

Claforan injection

Codeine sulfate

Cod liver oil

Coly-Mycin M Parenteral

Coly-Mycin S Oral Suspension

Comhist LA Capsule

Compazine Syrup

Cortenema (hydrocortisone retention enema)

Cortril hydrocortisone topical ointment

Dallergy Syrup

Dantrium Intravenous

Debrox Drops

DHE 45 Injection

DiaBeta Tablets

Diapid Nasal Spray

Dilantin-30/Pediatric Dilantin-125

Dilor G Liquid and Tablets

Dimetane Ten

Ditropan Syrup
Docusate Sodium Capsules
Docusate Sodium with
    Casanthranol Capsules
Dopram Injectable

Elase
Emcyt Capsules
Endep Tablets
Entex LA Tablets
Entex Liquid
Equagesic Tablets

Festal II Digestive Aid Tablets
Festalan Tablets
Flagyl I.V.
Flagyl I.V. RTU
Flagyl Tablets
Fluogen
Fumerin Tablets
Furacin Products-Topical Cream
Furadantin Oral Suspension
Furosemide Injection

Gantrisin Pediatric Suspension
Gantrisin Syrup
Gaviscon

Histatapp Elixir
Hydergine LC Liquid Capsules
Hydergine Oral Tablets,
    Sublingual Tablets, and
    Liquid

Ipsatol DM
Isordil Chewable Tablets
Isordil Tembids Capsules
Isordil Tembids Tablets
Isordil Titrados Tablets

Kie Syrup
Klor-Con Powder
Klor-Con 8/ Klor-Con 10
Klor-Con/25 Powder
Klor-10%
Klorvess Effervescent Granules
Klorvess Effervescent Tablets

Lactocal-F Tablets
Laraodopa Tablets
Lasix Oral Solution
Levsin Drops
Levsin Elixir
Levsin PB Drops
Levsin PB Elixir
Lidex (cream, gel, ointment,
    topical solution)
Lidex-E Cream
Lidex Ointment
Lidex Topical Solution
Lithonate Capsules
Lithotabs Tablets
Lomotil Tablets and Liquid

Medihaler-Epi
Medihaler Ergotamine Aerosol
Mestinon Syrup

Metamucil (powder contains dextrose)

Methergine Injection

Milk of magnesia

Mineral oil

Mycelex Troches

Mycostatin Oral Suspension

Mytrex Cream and Ointment

Nitr-o-Bid (IV, ointment, 2.5 plateau caps, 6.5 and 9 plateau caps)

Nitrostat Injection

Nitrostat Ointment 2%

Nitrostat Tablets

Nydrazid Syrup

Omnipen for Oral Suspension

Omnipen Pediatric Drops

Pamelor Solution

Penicillin G Potassium for Injections

Penicillin G Potassium Tablets

Pen Vee K Oral Solution

Pen Vee K Tablets

Pfizerpen-AS

Pfizerpen capsules and oral suspension

Pfizerpen VK tablets and oral suspension

Polymyxin B Sulfate

Procan SR

Prolixin Decanoate

Prolixin Elixir

Prolixin Enanthate

Prompt

Reglan Injectable

Rid (topical)

RMS (suppositories) Uniserts

Robaxin Injectable

Robicillin for VK Oral Solution

Robinul Injectable

Rocaltrol Tablets

Roniscol Timespan Tablets

Saccharin tablets

Secobarbital Sodium Capsules

Silvadene Cream (topical)

Sinarest 12 Hour Nasal Spray

SK Chloral Hydrate Capsules

SK Potassium Chloride Oral Solution

Sorbitol

Star-Otic

Stelazine Concentrate

Stoxil Ophthalmic Ointment

Stoxil Ophthalmic Solution

Streptase

Streptomycin Sulfate

Sumycin Syrup

Surmontil Capsules

Sweeta Liquid

Synacort Cream

Synalar HP Cream

Synalar Ointment

Synalgos DC Capsules

Syntocinon Injection

Syntocinon Nasal Spray

Tagamet Liquid

Terra Cortril Opthalmic
  Suspension

Terra Cortril Topical Ointment

Terramycin IM

Terramycin Ophthalmic
  Ointment

Theo-Dur Sprinkle

Theo-24 Capsules

Theolair-Plus Liquid

Theolair-Plus Tablets

Theragran Liquid

Thorazine Concentrate

Thorazine Syrup

Topicort Cream

Topicort Gel

Topicycline

Trecator-SC Tablets

Tuss-Ornade Liquid

Tylenol Children's Chewable
  Tablets

Urolene Blue

Urtex

Vi Penta F Chewables

Vi Penta F Drops

Virilon

Vistaril

Wygesic Tablets

Wymox Capsules

Wymox Oral Suspension

Yeast tablets

Yeast X

Zantac

Zaroxolyn Tablets

Foods Containing High Oxalic Acid

Beans in tomato sauce

Beets

Blackberries

Black raspberries

Blueberries

Celery

Chocolate

Cocoa

Collards

Concord grapes

Dandelion greens

Eggplant

Escarole

Green gooseberries

Green peppers

Grits

Lager beer

Leeks

Lemon peel

Lime peel

Okra

Parsley

Peanuts

Pecans

Red currants

Rhubarb

Soybean crackers

Spinach

Summer squash

Sweet potatoes

Swiss chard

Tea

Wheat germ

Resources for a Green Home Environment for Healthy Living

Natural Organic Body, Beauty, and Health Care Products

Bare Escentuals
Bare Escentuals Cosmetics
www.bareescentuals.com
71 Stevenson Street, 22nd Floor
San Francisco, CA 94105
415-489-5000
800-227-3990

*Burt's Bees Inc.
www.burtsbees.com
Attn: Customer Care
P.O. Box 13489
Durham, NC 27709
866-422-8787

Canus Goats Milk Company
www.canusgoatsmilk.com
5 Pilgrim Park
Waterbury, Vermont 05676
802-244-4628

Daniel Field Products
(natural hair color)
www.danielfield.com
Daniel Field Products, Ltd.
P.O. Box 591
Rotherham
S66 3WS
England

Honesty Cosmetics
www.honestycosmetics.co.uk
Lumford Mill, Bakewell
Derbyshire
DE45 1GS
England
01629-814-888

Mountain Rose Herbs
www.mountainroseherbs.com
P.O. Box 50220
Eugene, OR 97405
800-879-3337

Organic Universe, Inc.
www.organicuniverse.com
P.O. Box 4018
Wantagh, NY 11793
516-221-1600
info@organicuniverse.com

Purely Shea
www.purelyshea.com
6260 East Riverside Blvd., # 196
Loves Park, IL 61111
877-ORG-SHEA

Super Natural Mom
www.supernaturalmom.com

*Terressentials
www.terressentials.com
2650 Old National Pike
Middletown, MD 21769-8817
301-371-7333

*Tom's of Maine
www.tomsofmaine.com
Tom's of Maine
Consumer Dialogue Department
302 Lafayette Center
Kennebunk, ME 04043
800-367-8667
207-985-2944

Natural Household Cleaners

Citrus Magic
www.citrusmagic.com

Drugstore.com
www.drugstore.com

Ecover Power of Nature
www.ecover.com/us/en
800-449-4925

Natural Cleaning
www.ezinfocenter.com/26700/
showIndex.vstore

Our Green House
www.ourgreenhouse.com
Our Green House
365 South Main Street
Newtown, CT 06470
203-364-1484

Sun and Earth
www.sunandearth.com

Online Organic Food Resources

www.diamondorganics.com

www.graigfarm.co.uk/website.htm

*My personal favorites

Water Filters

Most of our sources of drinking water, including municipal water systems, wells, lakes, rivers, and even glaciers, contain some level of contamination. Contaminants range from naturally occurring minerals to man-made chemicals and by-products. While many contaminants are found at levels low enough to cause no immediate discomfort or sickness, low-level exposure to many common contaminants can, over time, cause severe illnesses, including liver damage, cancer, and other serious ailments. Even the chemicals commonly used to treat municipal water supplies, such as chlorine and fluoride, can be toxic and are known to have significant adverse effects on the human body. People with asthma and sensitivities should be particularly careful about additional exposure to toxins, and some people are even sensitive to the substances found in water itself, including substances inherent to the area from which the water came, the pH, and the water's plastic container.

Water filters are an easy and efficient way to remove these impurities from our drinking water. There are many types of water filters, and each has advantages and disadvantages. The two main types used in the household are charcoal water filters and reverse osmosis water filters.

Be aware that whatever type of filter you choose is only as good as its installation and maintenance. All filters require maintenance and periodic replacement of the filter media, membranes, or other parts, depending on the type of filter.

CHARCOAL WATER FILTERS

The charcoal used in water filters is derived from coconut husks. It readily absorbs impurities as the water passes along its surface area. The charcoal can be ground into small pieces or formed into a solid, yet porous, block in order to increase its surface area for attaching toxins. Charcoal water filters comprise possibly 95 percent of those in use domestically because they are simple to install, relatively economical, and effectively remove many toxins found in the environment. The filter's effectiveness depends on the charcoal's rating. According to the EPA, charcoal filters must be rated to remove particles one micron or larger to effectively remove the most deadly contaminants, cryptosporidium and giardia. Charcoal filters are particularly good at removing volatile organic compounds (VOCs) and particulates. However, they usually do not remove minerals in solution.

REVERSE OSMOSIS WATER FILTERS

The process of reverse osmosis was developed as a water treatment method more than forty years ago. This process first arose as a technique for desalinating seawater. Once the method's decontaminating capabilities were recognized, reverse osmosis systems began to be commercially produced for home water-purification purposes. Such systems were installed in homes as early as the 1970s.

The reverse osmosis process depends upon a semipermeable membrane through which pressurized water is forced. Reverse osmosis, simply stated, is the opposite of water's natural osmosis process. Osmosis is the name for water's tendency to migrate from a weaker saline solution to a stronger saline solution, gradually equalizing the saline composition of each solution when a semipermeable membrane separates the two solutions. In reverse osmosis, water is forced to move from a stronger saline solution to a weaker solution, again through a semipermeable membrane. Because salt molecules are physically larger than water molecules, the membrane blocks the passage of salt particles. The end result is desalinated water on one side of the membrane and a highly concentrated saline solution of water on the other side. In addition to salt particles, this process will remove a select number of drinking water contaminants, depending upon the physical size of the contaminants. However, while better at filtering dissolved minerals than charcoal filters, reverse osmosis filters are not as good at removing some VOCs since these substances are often small enough to pass directly through the membrane.

COMBINATION FILTERS

There are now a number of commercially available water filters that combine the advantages of both charcoal and reverse osmosis. Many come with three filters: a sediment filter, a charcoal filter, and a reverse osmosis filter. This combination combines the advantages of each and delivers relatively pure and good-tasting water.

There are other water purification devices, but charcoal and reverse osmosis are the most common in the household. A brief description of some other water purification devices follows. These filters are known for their convenience; however, they do not operate on the same principles as true filters.

WATER DISTILLER FILTERS

Water distillers use electricity to heat tap water to its boiling point. Impurities are left in the boiling container, and the purified condensate drains back into a clean container. These types of systems require a fair degree of power and cannot provide an immediate water supply because the boiling process must be completed before the water becomes available. There are now a number of reports that distilled water is not good to drink long term because it leaches nutrients from the body. However, this may be a good temporary solution for hypersensitive people.

IONIZED WATER FILTERS

Ionized water is electronically enhanced water that has been run over positive and negative electrodes and become ionized by separating the water and the minerals it contains into 70 percent alkaline and 30 percent acidic water. The alkaline ionized water is used for drinking and demonstrates strong antioxidant effects on the body, while the acidic ionized water is used on the outside of the body and has been proven to kill many types of bacteria, including E. coli.

ULTRAVIOLET WATER FILTERS

Ultraviolet water filters use a UV light to kill bacteria in the water. They are seldom seen in homes because of the difficulty in keeping the light clean. Some water ionizers are fitted with small UV lights, but these often have little or no effect. When working properly, ultraviolet light is very effective in killing bacteria but does not remove dissolved minerals, particulates, or VOCs.

Air Filters

Reducing exposure to allergens and irritants that are suspended in air can often help to reduce sensitivities and asthma symptoms. Air filters (also called air cleaners) and other air-purifying devices are the way to do this.

Common airborne particles range in size from .001 to 100 microns. A micron is about one twenty-five thousandth of an inch. To get an idea of size, a hair from your head is about 250 microns in diameter. Your body can only filter the larger contaminants, above 10 microns in size. A regular furnace filter removes some other contaminants. Problems can occur when smaller particles are present or when someone is unusually sensitive to a particular contaminant. Smaller airborne particles such as tobacco smoke and fine household dust can enter the deeper parts of the lungs. Air cleaners remove some but not all particles from the air.

There are numerous types of air cleaning systems, all with advantages and disadvantages in terms of cost, maintenance required, and effectiveness. Your choices should be determined by your budget and the severity of your allergies. Two websites for more information on filters are www.filters-now.com/ld3mspec.php and www.natlallergy.com/Default.asp?bhcd2=1152769454.

Air cleaners can be divided into two basic groups: portable or tabletop models, and those you install with, or in place of, an existing furnace and air conditioner filter.

PORTABLE AIR CLEANERS

Portable air cleaners are made to clean air in smaller areas, not in the whole house. Air cleaners usually use filters, electrical attraction, or ozone to remove small particles from the air.

The filters in some portable air cleaners trap particles. The finer the filter, the smaller the particles it traps. HEPA (high-efficiency particulate arresting) filters are the best. They can capture up to 99 percent of particles down to 0.3 microns in size. But gas molecules, which include radon and tobacco smoke, are extremely small and can pass through a HEPA filter. An activated carbon or charcoal filter usually is added to trap gas molecules.

Pleated (also called "media") filters use materials like the HEPA filters, but they capture fewer particles because they are not packed as tightly. They are 40 to 95 percent effective and remove most household dust.

Electronic cleaners use electrical attraction. This type of cleaner uses electrostatic precipitation, static charge, or particle ionization to remove particles drawn in by a fan through a foam prefilter. Larger particles are trapped at this point. Particles are then charged by a high-voltage wire and captured in the precipitating cell. A carbon filter removes odors, and a postfilter removes other particles.

When a prefilter is used, the electrostatic precipitator can remove mold, bacteria, tobacco smoke, and most household dust. Regular maintenance is a must.

A negative ionizer also uses a foam prefilter and a carbon filter. It is unique because it has charged wires, which create ions. The fan blows these ions into the air, and traps the charged particles (chemicals, bacteria, and allergens) using an electrostatic charge.

An ozone generator is a type of air cleaner that uses a high-voltage electrical charge to change oxygen to ozone. High concentrations of ozone can destroy gas molecules and some microorganisms, such as mold spores. However, there is considerable agreement that overexposure to ozone can be harmful, so these types of cleaners are best used in basements or other unoccupied areas for mold remediation or odor removal. The U.S. Environmental

Protection Agency does not recommend these for occupied areas, such as bedrooms, where there are long exposures.

In-duct air cleaners are designed to fit into a house's heating and air-conditioning system ductwork or air-conditioning unit. Standard fiber filters can be used, the kind found in most standard air-conditioning units. These typically have very little ability to remove small particles and are designed primarily to protect the air-conditioning unit coils from becoming clogged.

Pleated (media) filters are more efficient than the standard fiber filters. Recently the American Society of Heating Refrigeration and Air Conditioning Engineers (ASHRAE) and the air filter industry have come up with a standardized rating system, based on the European concept, of a MERV (minimum efficiency reporting value) rating for each type of air filter. The higher the MERV rating, the greater the air filter's efficiency. This numbering system makes it easier to evaluate and compare mechanical air filters and will hopefully eliminate some of the confusion regarding the overall effectiveness of any type of mechanical air filter on removing airborne particulates, especially those that are less than two microns in size.

MERV ratings for several air filters follow:

+ Throw-Away Fiberglass Media: MERV 1–4

+ Pleated Media Air Filters, 30 percent ASHRAE grade media: MERV 10–11

+ Pleated Media Air Filters, 65 percent ASHRAE grade media: MERV 13 (65 percent ASHRAE grade media is about 20 percent effective on particles smaller than 1 micron)

+ Pleated Media Air Filters, 95 percent: MERV 14

HEPA filters, which are available for in-duct air cleaners, exceed these efficiencies and are rated differently. However, HEPA filters are not practical for home air-conditioning units due to their large pressure-drop requirements. Charcoal filters can also be highly effective in screening out particulates and can also remove gaseous contaminants. However, these also have high pressure drops, making them impractical to use with a standard air-conditioning unit fan.

Electrostatic filters can be used to replace a standard furnace filter. An electrostatic filter installed in the return air duct near the furnace removes finer particles from the air. These can sometimes be highly effective, depending on their rating. However, the more effective they are, the more often they will need to be replaced.

ELECTRONIC AIR CLEANERS

Electronic air cleaners use a series of wires in a grid form that are electrically charged. These charged wires (or plates in some units) attract the particles being drawn in by the heating and cooling fan. There is no media in which the particles can be trapped and no additional dust cake for continued air filtration efficiency. Every time the wires or plates are charged, they loosen some of the particles that are attached. Thus, as the wires become coated, the electronic air cleaner system's efficiency is reduced. In fact, an electronic air cleaner is the only air-filtering device that becomes less efficient as it loads up. Its efficiency can start out as a MERV 12 but drop down to a MERV 8 rating within one week of operation. As a result of their type of performance, they do not use a MERV rating. Electronic air cleaner units need to be cleaned frequently to maintain good efficiency.

UV Lights

Ultraviolet lights (germicidal lamps), or UV systems, come in both "hot plasma" (8,000 hours of life) and "cold plasma" (36,000 hours of life) lamp systems. They produce a specific wavelength of 253 nanometers and produce UV C. This C wavelength has the ability to affect microbiological contaminants such as mold and bacteria. The UV C light can destroy the contaminant's DNA and keep it from replicating. UV C has no effect on solid particles, and it does *not* remove anything from the airstream. UV C lights are normally placed in the return airstream, although the speed of the air past the lights can minimize the UV lights' effectiveness. These UV lights can be very useful when placed within an air conditioner to shine on the cooling coils and drain pans, as the light can irradiate these moist areas all the time and help minimize the growth of mold or bacteria. UV lights are an ancillary piece of equipment and should always be used in conjunction with an air filter or air filtration system.

BioSET Resources

DETOXIFICATION REGIMES:

Please refer to the detoxification questionnaire in *The Food Allergy Cure* by Ellen W. Cutler, DC.

TO ORDER ENZYME PRODUCTS
AND DETOXIFICATION REMEDIES:

+ Excellent-quality vegetarian enzymes, homeopathic remedies for detoxification, empty glass vials, and copies of Dr. Cutler's books, CDs, and video can be ordered at (877) 927-0741 or www.bioset.net.

  + The *Creating Wellness* videotape gives a clear step-by-step demonstration of the BioSET Food Allergy Home Clearing described in chapter 10.
  + The BioSET Food Allergen Kit provides twenty-four vials containing over two hundred common food sensitivities. Empty vials are also available for preparing your food sensitivities that are not provided in the kit.
  + Remedies for drainage, detoxification, energy production, and specific organ support include Drainage, Detox, Recharge, Bladder Cleanse, Blood Cleanse, Colon Cleanse, Kidney Cleanse, Liver Cleanse, Lung Cleanse, Lymph Cleanse, Skin Cleanse, Small Intestine Cleanse, and Spleen Cleanse.
  + Enzyme supplements aid with digestive and system balance.

CONSUMER WORKSHOPS AND PROFESSIONAL SEMINARS:

BioSET provides information for the public and professionals, and referrals to practitioners trained in this method, as well as workshops and seminars. The BioSET website also provides a complete up-to-date list of all the certified BioSET practitioners worldwide.

The BioSET Institute

www.bioset.net
116 E. Blithedale Avenue
Mill Valley, CA 94941
Phone: (877) 927-0741 or (415) 384-0200
Fax: (415) 384-0199

New Research on Asthma and Respiratory Disease

While it is peripheral to the BioSET system, the following research might be of interest to people with asthma.

Asthma and Foods

Much research has been done on the link between a person's diet and their asthmatic symptoms.

ADULTS ON A SPECIAL FOOD DIET

By Dr. Gus Borok, a medical doctor in South Africa, decided to conduct an asthma trial in private practice. He recruited asthma patients via the media, radio talks, press advertisements, and advertisements on posters. Professor J. M. Loots, previously of the Pretoria University Sports Research Centre, performed the original lung function tests; if volunteers satisfied conditions that classified them as asthmatic, he randomized them into control groups and groups on a special food program. Of the 102 asthmatics recruited for the trial, half were put on the special diet, and the other half simply continued under their own doctor's care with no lifestyle changes.

Professor Loots repeated the lung function tests weekly with both groups for six weeks. The lung function of the group on the special food program improved by 21 percent, whereas the control group improved by only 1.8 percent. After six weeks, twenty-seven members of the control group decided to go on the diet, after which their lung function improved by a further

20 percent. The results demonstrated that 70 percent of asthma attacks were due to foods only, 20 percent were due to the combination of a food and an inhalant, and 10 percent were due to inhalants only.

After being on the special diet for several weeks, of the seventy-eight patients who used various inhaled bronchodilator medications, only seventeen needed to use this medication when they accidentally ate a processed food containing an asthma trigger. Similarly, of the sixty-seven patients on the special diet who used oral or inhaled corticosteroids, only eight needed this therapy after avoiding all foods listed by the special food program as asthma triggers.

None of these patients were instructed to discontinue their traditional therapy. However, some individuals found that they no longer needed their medications once they had changed their diet. One patient no longer needed to receive monthly injections of cortisone. Eight out of ten patients who used nebulizer inhalation therapy no longer needed this drug. All patients who used fenoterol, ipratropium bromide, and fenoterol/ipratropium no longer required this therapy, with the exception of two cases of individuals who used these drugs in an emergency.

Smoking played a minor role in the study. Of the 102 asthmatics, more than half (sixty-nine individuals) had never smoked, twenty-one had stopped smoking, and only twelve still smoked. In eight patients, passive cigarette smoke triggered wheezing.

The trigger foods involved in the study (to be avoided by participants) were the following:

+ Fruits: apples, pears, bananas, citrus, and melons
+ Vegetables: avocados, potatoes, tomatoes, and onions
+ Spices: triggers in only three cases
+ Nuts: walnuts, almonds, and cashews; triggers in only five cases
+ Proteins: milk products; milk itself was the most common trigger, followed by cheese, yogurt, and feta cheese
+ Proteins: beef was a more common trigger than any other animal or bird protein
+ Grains: wheat (including cakes and cookies made with wheat), bread, and pasta were the most common triggers; next came maize (corn), followed by rice and oats
+ Processed foods: triggers in fourteen instances only
+ Beverages: played the smallest role; wine was the most common trigger, followed by beer, fruit juices, coffee, tea, and in one instance only, tomato sauce[1]

CHILDREN ON AN ELIMINATION AND ROTATION DIET

A pediatric pulmonologist randomly organized sixty children aged six months to twelve years into a special diet group and a control group. The thirty children in the control group were kept on therapy for asthma, and the remaining thirty subjects were placed on an elimination and rotation diet. He then assessed the severity of asthma in both groups before and after the trial period of six weeks. During this period, the special diet group's food intake was carefully monitored.

In the special diet group, twenty-five out of thirty children experienced relief in their asthma symptoms without the need for any therapy. Of the remaining five, four went on reduced therapy, needing only 50 mcg of cortisone inhalants once daily, instead of their usual 250 mcg twice daily. Only one patient showed no improvement. All thirty children in the control group continued to need therapy to control their asthma.

After six weeks, those in the special diet group who had not significantly improved were tested for environmental factors known to cause asthma. Five of the children were found to be sensitive to inhalants as well as foods.

The trigger foods involved in the study (to be avoided by participants) were

+ Proteins: milk and milk products (seventeen instances) and beef (three), were the main triggers, followed by chicken and eggs (one each)

+ Fruits and vegetables (nine instances total): squash family (two) and apple, banana, paw-paw, potato, tomato, beans, and soya (one each)

+ Grains: bread and wheat (nine) and maize (one)

+ Processed foods (eleven instances total): chocolate (three), potato chips (two), and Liqui Fruit fruit juice, ice cream, tomato crisps, slush puppies (fruit and crushed ice beverages), and carry-out chicken and hamburger (one each); all of these processed foods contain either milk, wheat, fruit, or a protein that were among the trigger foods

+ Preservatives: only one child's asthma was triggered by foods containing preservatives

Follow-up studies done one to two years later showed that, aside from the four children on reduced therapy, four other children who had originally reacted to foods needed therapy only when they ate foods that triggered their symptoms.[2]

BREAST-FED INFANTS WHOSE MOTHERS WENT ON AN ELIMINATION AND ROTATION DIET

The mothers of twelve breast-fed infants were placed on an elimination and rotation diet. (This is very significant; I have found that when mothers avoid the foods to which they are sensitive, their children have less respiratory symptoms.) The purpose of this program was to identify whether any foods in the mothers' diets or any environmental factors triggered asthma symptoms (such as mucus on the chest, cough, and/or rib retraction) in their infants. Unfortunately, no controls were considered for a crossover survey.

Eleven of the twelve infants were symptom-free when their mother avoided the triggers. Only one infant showed no improvement.

The trigger foods involved in the study (to be avoided by participants) were

+ Protein: cow's milk (six instances)

+ Grains: wheat (two)

+ Chocolate, wine, and citrus (one each)

+ Miscellaneous: besides cow's milk, an inhalant (the mother's perfume) made one infant's symptoms worse[3]

FISH OIL

BioSET practitioners recommend fish oil for many immune disorders, including asthma, and the research backs this up.

Fish Oil and Exercise-Induced Asthma

New research has shown that adding fish oil supplements to their diet can help prevent the constriction of airways in asthmatics who suffer exercise-induced asthma. A recent study performed by Dr. Timothy D. Mickleborough from Indiana University in Bloomington demonstrated that fish oil supplements can improve lung function in elite athletes (highly skilled athletes who have been participating in a sport for a significant period of time) who suffered from asthma. The results suggested that fish oil's anti-inflammatory properties were the active agent causing the positive effects.

This study assessed the athletes' pre- and post-exercise lung function along with inflammatory markers in their sputum following an exercise-induced asthma attack. For three weeks, one group of athletes was given a normal diet supplemented with fish oil capsules. The control group was given a placebo. Then after a two-week interval, during which no supplements were given, the participants switched groups.

During the period of time when they were following a normal diet supplemented only with a placebo, individuals in each group developed asthma when exercising. However, when study participants were in the groups supplemented with fish oil, they experienced a noticeable decrease in asthma. In fact, their respiratory response was not even in the range clinically diagnosed as exercise-induced asthma. The fish oil supplements also caused a significant drop in inflammatory markers in the sputum. Participants received twenty capsules of fish oil per day.[4]

Fish Oil and Asthma in Children

In 1994–1995, researchers at the Department of Pediatrics of the National Higashi Saitama Hospital in Japan conducted a fish oil study involving eighty asthmatic children. Over a ten-month period, the patients in this study all received the same foods and exposure to the same inhaled allergens. The researchers found that dietary supplementation with fish oil rich in omega-3 and the polyunsaturated fatty acids EPA and DHA decreased asthma scores for the children.

Of the active ingredients in the fish oil capsules, the omega-3 fatty acids reduce the generation of immune mediators from inflammatory cells, and EPA is known to inhibit the formation of leukotrienes from arachidonic acids, or immune mediators (thus reducing inflammation). The data therefore suggest that supplementation with fish oil for ten months improved airway inflammation.[5]

A NEW DIET FOR ASTHMATICS

Scientists claim to have discovered a new diet that not only supports weight loss, but can also help people with asthma. Dr. James Johnson, who cowrote the report with colleagues from Stanford and New Orleans universities, reports that the diet consists of eating normally one day, then cutting food intake to between 20 and 50 percent the next day.

Dr. Johnson lost thirty-five pounds during the first eleven weeks he was on the diet. Within two weeks, he also noticed an improvement in a variety of disease conditions, including his asthma. There has been some scientific speculation that this food program may also have a positive impact on people suffering from insulin resistance, rheumatoid arthritis, and multiple sclerosis.[6]

Vitamin C and Asthma

A recent study conducted by the Medical Research Council at Cambridge and published in the scientific journal *Thorax* suggests that a deficiency of vitamin C and of the mineral manganese may contribute to adult asthma. The vitamin C deficiency appears to be primarily associated with a diet that is deficient in fruit.

This study showed that a moderate consumption of vitamin C, equivalent to half an orange or less per day, decreased the risk of asthma by 12 percent, and a higher fruit consumption, more than half an orange or a fourth of a grapefruit per day, decreased the risk by 41 percent.[7]

Asthma and Antioxidants

Lisa Wood, a research fellow at the Respiratory and Sleep Medicine Unit of the Hunter Medical Research Institute, associated with the University of Newcastle in New South Wales, led a study on the effect of diets low in anti-oxidants. These Australian researchers confirmed that diets low in antioxidants, especially those low in the tomato pigment lycopene, can worsen asthma attacks.

In a study involving fourteen asthma sufferers (since expanded to twenty-four), asthmatic subjects were monitored while on a low-antioxidant diet. Almost three-quarters of the volunteers had lower levels of antioxidants in their blood due to this diet. After ten days, the asthma symptoms of those with lower levels of lycopene had gotten worse.[8]

Immune Cells in Asthmatics

In the *New England Journal of Medicine*, March 2006 issue, it was reported that the immune system cells that cause asthma might be natural killer (NK) T cells. Dr. Dale Umetsu, a professor of pediatrics at Harvard Medical School and Children's Hospital Boston, and Jonathan Field, a visiting professor at Stanford University in California, conducted this study. They concluded, "The majority of T cells in people with asthma aren't what we thought they were."

Natural killer T cells were only recently discovered because the technology for this type of research is very new, explains Dr. Umetsu. T cells, part of the immune system, help fight foreign invaders such as bacteria and viruses. In asthma, the immune cells become a bit chaotic and don't work as they should, instead producing an inflammatory reaction.

Studies on natural killer T cells were conducted on samples taken from fourteen people with asthma, comparing them to samples from six healthy controls and five people with another inflammatory lung disorder called sarcoidosis, which is unrelated to asthma.

About 60 percent of the T cells in the asthma group were not the expected helper T cells, which had previously been thought to be the case. Instead, they were natural killer T cells. Neither the healthy control group nor the people with sarcoidosis had natural killer T cells in their samples.

As far as the researchers know, none of the current asthma therapies are focused on targeting natural killer T cells. Umetsu said that researchers have to learn more about how these cells work and what initially causes them to go into the lungs. Natural killer T cells are a very different type of immune cell and appear to respond to different substances than helper T cells.[9]

Risk of Asthma for Children Living On or Near Livestock Farms

A study conducted at the University of Iowa found that large-scale livestock farms located near schools may pose a risk of asthma to children. Concentrated animal-feeding operations seem to release inflammatory substances that can affect not only the health of workers at these operation facilities, but also the quality of air in nearby communities. Studies have shown that there is an increased rate of asthma in children living in these types of rural areas.

Researchers collected data from the parents of kindergarten through fifth-grade students attending two Iowa elementary schools. One of these schools was located half a mile from a concentrated animal-feeding operation, and the other school was more than ten miles away.

The study, which was published in *Chest*, found that the prevalence rate for physician-diagnosed asthma was 24.6 percent at the school close to the facility compared to 11.7 percent at the control school.[10]

Asthma and the Workplace

As many as one in ten Australians who develop asthma as an adult seem to blame it on their workplace. New statistics released in Australia show that hairdressers, spray painters, and other people with chemical-related jobs are at greater risk of developing asthma than average.

This research was conducted at the Woolcock Medical Institute in Sydney on 3,300 eighteen- to forty-nine-year-olds who filled out and returned a mailed questionnaire.

The study focused on finding a link between asthma and exposure to conditions experienced in a range of occupations known to be at risk for occupational asthma. They discovered that 9.5 percent of adult-onset asthmatics developed asthma after working in a "high-risk" job. Dr. Guy Marks, head of epidemiology at the Woolcock Institute, said the occupations were varied, including automotive repair, electronics manufacturing, farm work, bakeries, hairdressing, the pharmaceutical industry, dry cleaners, printers, and people working with laboratory animals. Even health care workers are at risk because they regularly use gloves made of latex, known to cause sensitivity reactions. Marks said employers are obliged to do all they can to control exposure to this irritant if possible.[11]

Perfumes and Chemicals Banned in Canada

Politicians in the city of Ottawa in Canada are considering a program to get people to stop using perfume, scented soaps, cleaners, and deodorants—to possibly ban them altogether in public places. The people behind this program feel that more and more people are becoming sensitive to the chemicals used to make scents, and many of these chemicals have been known to trigger asthma attacks. The ban would be in effect in all city buildings, on public transportation, and in sports and community centers. It is even under consideration to have the ban include bars, restaurants, malls, and all workplaces. Politicians are also considering a campaign to switch from scented cleaning products to unscented ones in public places.

This program is based on an effort to promote wellness, reduce sick time, and provide a healthy work environment. Of course, strong reactions are expected from the fragrance industry and from people who want to use perfumes and scented products. If Ottawa passed a law against scents, it would be the first place in Canada to do so. Other anti-scent public campaigns are under way in Nova Scotia and in the city of Halifax.[12]

Treatments: Exercise the Lungs

Australian researchers report that in some cases, lung exercises can help people with mild asthma cut back on the amount of medication they need to control their condition. In a study involving fifty-seven adults, researchers found that the use of reliever inhalers dropped by more than 80 percent, based on exercising the lung with specific exercises. About half the group used a technique calling for shallow nasal breathing with slow exhalations. The other half used a technique based on upper body exercises alternating with relaxation. Both groups were instructed to try to do the exercises before taking their medication.

The authors of this study stated, "The similarity of the improvements seen in both groups, despite the widely disparate nature of the breathing exercises they were using, suggests that the observed changes were more likely to be attributable to one or more of the shared *process* elements—such as the instruction to use the exercises initially in place of a reliever for symptom relief—than to the breathing exercises themselves."[13]

Asthma Medication and Cataracts

Some studies have suggested that asthma drugs can play a role in causing cataracts in seniors. Researchers at McGill University Health Centre in Montreal, Canada, and epidemiologist Sammy Suissa claim that seniors who regularly use inhalers with cortisone-based medication should switch to other forms of treatment. Otherwise, they could face a risk of developing severe cataracts.

Sammy Suissa's team studied provincial health data for one hundred thousand patients, with an average age of seventy-eight, over a fourteen-year period. With these patients, who used a cortisone-based inhaler drug for asthma for at least four years, researchers saw a 24 percent jump in the number who developed cataracts. The risk was high when even half the drug's dose was used. Suissa suggests using other medication instead, possibly bronchodilators that open the bronchial tubes.[14]

Alternative Remedies for Asthma

Multiple studies via peer-reviewed journals have established and validated the anti-asthma properties of the metabolites magnesium, pyridoxine (vitamin B6), and cobalamin (vitamin B12), and the herbs *Coleus forskholi* and *Ginkgo biloba*.

Pyridoxine, or vitamin B6, is a critical coenzyme in human biochemistry. Both pyridoxine and magnesium mediate metabolic processes such as producing adenosine triphosphate (ATP) and cyclic adenosine monophosphate (cAMP). ATP and cAMP have been shown to help relax bronchial smooth muscle tissue, resulting in an increase of airway circumference. Vitamin B6 also plays a critical role in the utilization of various amino acids, such as L-tryptophan and L-tyrosine and is, therefore, the key coenzyme in synthesizing neurotransmitters such as serotonin, adrenaline, and norepinephrine.

Many medications have been demonstrated to potentially cause a deficiency of pyridoxine, which might exacerbate asthma symptoms. Some of these pharmaceutical agents include theophylline (an oral methylxanthine), albuterol (an inhaled beta-adrenergic agonist), and prednisone (an oral steriod form of cortisone).

In several nutritional articles, supplementation with cobalamin (vitamin B12) has been demonstrated to improve the symptoms of asthma overall by reducing its severity and frequency. Jonathan V. Wright, MD, of Kent, Washington, believes that vitamin B12 therapy is especially helpful for childhood asthma because it has been shown to produce a sulfite-cobalamin complex that can block the allergic effects of sulfites.[15]

The ginkgo tree has been planted throughout the United States primarily as an ornament, often as part of an urban landscape along roadsides. A single tree may easily reach the age of one thousand years, and this species is very resistant to insects, disease, and pollution. The traditional use of ginkgo in China has almost always been related to lung function, blood circulation, longevity, and/or mental performance.

To date, *Ginkgo biloba* is the most widely prescribed phyto-pharmaceutical (made from plants) in the world, with over two hundred published studies and abstracts validating the herb's efficacy. The herb is considered to be clinically helpful for cerebral vascular insufficiency, Raynaud's phenomenon (involving poor circulation), and asthma. All of these diseases have common components: a physiological need for an increase in microcirculation and a reduction of platelets and clotting.

Ginkgo's biologically active compounds occur primarily in its leaves and are classified as ginkgo-flavoneglycosides and terpenoids. The terpenoids have been demonstrated to increase microcirculation and reduce the inflammatory response.

Endnotes

Introduction

1. American Lung Association, "Epidemiology and Statistics Unit, Research and Program Services," *Trends in Asthma Morbidity and Mortality* (May 2005): 4.

Chapter 1

1. Mark T. O'Hollaren, interview by Helen Fosam, "Allergic Diseases—How Big Is the Problem? An Expert Interview with Mark T. O'Hollaren, MD; Part 1 of 3: Overview of Epidemiology and Prevalence," *Medscape*, April 24, 2006. http://www.medscape.com/viewarticle/524717.

2. E. Ferguson, H. J. Cassaday. "Theoretical Accounts of Gulf War Syndrome: From Environmental Toxins to Psychological, Neuroimmunology, and Neurodegeneration," *Behavioural Neurology* 13: 3–4. www.ehponline.org/members/2004/6881/6881

3. Devin J. Starlanyl. "Reactive Hypoglycemia (RHG), Insulin Resistance: FMS and CMP Perpetuating Factor," adapted from *Fibromyalgia and Myofascial Pain: A Survival Manual*, 2nd ed. Starlanyl and Copeland. Oakland, CA: New Harbinger, 2001.

4. Kristin Lueck, "The Dietary Migraine: How Food Can Cause Headaches," *Nutrition Bytes* 3, no. 1 (1997) article 3. http://repositories.cdlib.org/uclabiolchem/nutritionbytes/vol3/iss1/art3; Mary Beth Franklin, *"Contain the Migraine," Vitality on Demand (August 2, 2004)*. www.rmhonline.com/modules/SelfCareWellness/vitWellness.asp?wellID=1024.

Chapter 3

1. Christian Nordqvist, "Homeopathy Helps 70 Percent of Patients with Chronic Diseases, Six-Year Study," *Medical News Today* (November 23, 2005). http://www.medicalnewstoday.com/healthnews.php?newsid=34046.

2. Virgil V. Strang, *Essential Principles of Chiropractic* (Davenport, Iowa: Palmer College of Chiropractic, 1985).

3. Lai Xinsheng, "Observation on the Curative Effect of Acupuncture on Type 1 Allergic Diseases," *Journal of Traditional Chinese Medicine* 13, no. 4 (1993): 243.

Chapter 4

1. "Asthma Facts and Figures," *Asthma and Allergy Foundation of America*. www.aafa.org.

2. J. N. Tsanakas et al., "Free Running Asthma Screening Test," *Archives of Disease in Childhood* 63 (1988): 261–265. http://adc.bmj.com/cgi/content/abstract/archdischild%3b63/3/261.

3. California Sinus Institute. Balloon sinuplasty information webpage. www.calsinus.com/balloon-sinuplasty.htm.

4. Robert B. Meek, "Middle Ear, Eustachian Tube, Inflammation/Infection," *eMedicine* (March 22, 2006). www.emedicine.com/ent/topic207.htm.

Chapter 5

1. David L. Hahn, "Asthma and Infection." *Asthma Story* 1.1 (July 26, 2005). www.asthmastory.com/research/doctor.pdf.

2. Zhou Zhu et al., "Acidic Mammalian Chitinase in Asthmatic Th2 Inflammation and IL-13 Pathway Activation." *Science* 304, no. 5677 (June 2004): 1678–1682.

3. John M. James et al., "Safe Administration of the Measles Vaccine to Children Allergic to Eggs," *The New England Journal of Medicine* 332, no. 19 (May 11, 1995): 1262–1266. http://content.nejm.org/cgi/content/full/332/19/1262#R15.

4. National Vaccine Information Center. Homepage. www.909shot.com.

5. D. Jarvis et al., "The Association of Hepatitis A and Helicobacter Pylori with Sensitization to Common Allergens, Asthma and Hay Fever in a Population of Young British Adults," *Allergy* 59, no. 10 (2004):1063-1067.

6. "Food Allergies Linked to Ear Infections," *Science News* (October 8, 1994). http://www.highbeam.com/doc/1G1-15824121.html.

7. National Institute of Allergy and Infectious Diseases, "Asthma: A Concern for Minority Populations," *National Institutes of Health* (October 2001). http://www.niaid.nih.gov/factsheets/asthma.htm.

8. Public Education Committee, "Tips to Remember: Food Allergy," *American Academy of Allergy, Asthma, and Immunology.* www.aaaai.org/patients/publicedmat/tips/foodallergy.stm.

9. Julian Crane et al., "Increased House Dust Mite Allergen in Synthetic Pillows May Explain Increased Wheezing," *BMJ* 314 (1997): 1763, www.bmj.bmjjournals.com/cgi/content/full/314/7079/518, reported in J. Kahn, "Synthetic Pillows May Aggravate Asthma Symptoms," *Medical Tribune News Service* (1995).

10. T. W. Wong, "Household Gas Cooking: A Risk Factor for Respiratory Illnesses in Preschool Children," *Archives of Disease in Childhood* 89, no. 7, (July 2004): 631–636.

11. Sami Youakim, "Work-Related Asthma," *American Family Physician* (December 1, 2001). http://www.aafp.org/afp/20011201/1839.html.

12. "Preventing Asthma and Death from Diisocyanate Exposure," *DHHS (NIOSH)* Publication No. 96–111 (1996). www.cdc.gov/Niosh/asthma.html.

13. John R. Froines, "An Evaluation of the Scientific Peer-Reviewed Research and Literature on the Human Health Effects of MTBE, Its Metabolites, Combustion Products and Substitute Compounds," University of California, Davis. www.tsrtp.ucdavis.edu/mtberpt/vol2.pdf.

Chapter 6

1. Ellen Cutler, *MicroMiracles, Discover the Healing Power of Enzymes*. (New York: Rodale, 2005): 86–88.

2. *High-Salt Diet May Aggravate Asthma in Men*. California Center for Medical Consumers, Inc., Magazine Collection 73A3454 (1994).

3. Carole Palmer et al., "The Impact of Fluoride on Health," *American Dietetic Association* 105, no. 10 (October 2005): 1620–1628.

Chapter 7

1. Kevin Murray, "ACAAI Calls for Action to Control Risk of Potentially Life-Threatening Latex Allergy," *The American College of Allergy, Asthma and Immunology* (July 18, 1995). http://web.archive.org/web/20030221011024/http://allergy.mcg.edu/news/m3.html.

2. Douglas M. Bibus, Ralph T. Holman, and William J. Walsh, "Fatty Acid Profiles of Schizophrenic Phenotypes," 91st AOCS Annual Meeting and Expo San Diego, California (April 25–28, 2000).

3. The Townsend Letter Group. Autoimmune Disease and Women. *Townsend Letter for Doctors and Patients*. (May 2003).

4. Loretta Lanphler, "PMS, Menopause and Asthma: Is There A Connection?" *Allergy, Asthma and Silence Relief Resource Center*. www.allergies-asthma-sinus-relief.org/asthma/pms-menopause-asthma.php; R. J. Troisi et al., "Menopause, Postmenopausal Estrogen Preparations, and the Risk of Adult-Onset Asthma. A Prospective Cohort Study," *American Journal of Respiratory and Critical Care Medicine* 152(1995): 1182–1188.

5. Charlotte E. Grayson, ed., "Heartburn and Asthma," *MedicineNet.com with WebMD and The Cleveland Clinic*. www.medicinenet.com/script/main/art.asp?articlekey=43181#affect.

6. L. Bieolory and R. Gandi, "Asthma and Vitamin C," *Annals Allergy* 73 (1994): 89–96. Canadian Asthma Prevention Institute, www.asthmaworld.org/Citations.htm.

7. J. Britton, "Dietary Magnesium, Lung Function, Wheezing, and Airway Hyperreactivity in a Random Adult Population Sample," *Lancet* 344, no. 8919 (August 6, 1994): 357–362.; S. K. Sharma, Bhargava Anurag, and J. N. Pande, "Effect of Parenteral Magnesium Sulphate on Pulmonary Functions in Bronchial Asthma," *J. Asthma* 3, no. 2 (1994): 109–115.

8. Alan L. Miller, "The Etiologies, Pathophysiology, and Alternative/Complementary Treatment of Asthma," *Alternative Medicine Review* 6, no. 1 (2001): 39.

Chapter 8

1. Sue Pleming, "New Study Highlights Teen Cigarette Brands," *Reuters* (August 31, 2000). Excerpts posted on *Action on Smoking and Health*, www.no-smoking.org/sept00/09-01-00-1.html.

2. "Advice from Your Allergist . . . Pet Allergy," American College of Allergy, Asthma & Immunology. www.acaai.org/public/advice/pets.htm.

3. George D. Thurston and David V. Bates, "Air Pollution as an Underappreciated Cause of Asthma Symptoms," *JAMA* 290, no. 14 (October 8, 2003): 1915–1917.

Chapter 9

1. Ralph J. Luciani, "Direct Observation and Photography of Electroconductive Points on Human Skin," *Am. J. Acupuncture* 6, no.4 (October–December 1978): 311–317.

Chapter 11

1. Theresa Tamkins, "Adult-Onset Asthma May Be Allergic Reaction to Bacteria," *Medical Tribune* (Medscape, 1995).

2. Mayo Clinic Staff, "Antibiotics: Too Much of a Good Thing," *MayoClinic.com* (February 13, 2006). www.mayoclinic.com/health/antibiotics/FL00075.

Chapter 12

1. R. Fiasse et al., "Circulating Immune Complexes and Disease Activity in Crohn's Disease," *Gut* 19 (1978): 611–617.

2. E. Cutler, "Reduce Cravings and Lose Weight" in *MicroMiracles, Discover the Healing Power of Enzymes* (New York: Rodale, 2005): 86–88.

Chapter 13

1. F. Gazdik et al., "Decreased Levels of Coenzyme Q(10) in Patients with Bronchial Asthma," *Allergy* 57, no. 9 (September 2002): 811–814.

Chapter 14

1. American Lung Association, "Epidemiology and Statistics Unit, Research and Program Services," *Trends in Asthma Morbidity and Mortality* (May 2005): 4–5.

Appendix A

1. *Stedman's Medical Dictionary,* 26th ed. (Philadelphia: Lippincott, Williams & Wilkins, 1995).

2. PubMed, National Library of Medicine, National Institutes of Health. www.ncbi.nlm. nih.gov/PubMed/. Accessed March 2002.

3. Ibid.

4. Ibid.

5. *Merriam Third New International Dictionary*, Vol. 111. (*Encyclopedia Britannica, Inc.* 1986).

Appendix C

1. Gus Borok, "Improving Health: The Role of Foods in Asthma," *The South African Journal of Natural Medicine* 22: 355–362. http://www.naturalmedicine.co.za/sajnm_main/article.php?story=20060608105819137.

2. Ibid.

3. Ibid.

4. Anthony J. Brown, "Fish Oil Can Prevent Airway Constriction in Asthma," *Reuters Health* (January 9, 2006).

5. T. Nagukura et al., "Dietary Supplementation with Fish Oil Rich in Omega-3 Poly-unsaturated Fatty Acids in Children with Bronchial Asthma," *Eur Respire J* 16 (2000): 861–865; M. Okamoto et al., "Immunology Effects of Perilla Seed Oil Supplementation on Leukotriene Generation by Leucocytes in Patients with Asthma Associated with Lipometabolism," *Int Arch Allergy Immunology* 122, no. 2 (June 2000): 137–42.

6. Roger Dobson, "Doctors Devise New Diet that Can Help Asthma and Arthritis," *The Independent on Sunday* (June 18, 2006).

7. B. D. Patel et al., "Dietary Antioxidants and Asthma in Adults," *Thorax* 61 (2006): 388–393.

8. "Diet Low in Antioxidants Tied to Worsened Asthma Attacks," *Health* (June 7, 2006). http://www.macleans.ca/topstories/health/article.jsp?content=20060601 _122442_4932#.

9. Omid Akbari et al., "CD4+ Invariant T-Cell–Receptor+ Natural Killer T Cells in Bronchial Asthma," *New England Journal of Medicine* 354, no. 11: 1117–1129, reported by Serena Gordon, "Immune System Cells May Be Cause of Asthma," *HealthDay News* (March 15, 2006). http://www.healthfinder.gov/news/newsstory. asp?docID=531583.

10. Sigurdur T. Sigurdarson and Joel N. Kline, "School Proximity to Concentrated Animal Feeding Operations and Prevalence of Asthma in Students," *Chest* 129 (June 2006): 1486–1491, reported in "Concentrated Animal Feeding Operations Near Schools May Pose Asthma Risk," *Medical News Today* with University of Iowa Health Science Relations (June 23, 2006).

11. Anthony Johnson et al., "Occupational Asthma in New South Wales (NSW): A Population-Based Study," *Occupational Medicine* 56, no. 4 (2006): 258–262, reported in "1 in 10 adults develop asthma at their workplace," *AZoMED.com*.

12. Jake Rupert, "City of Ottawa May Regulate Use of Perfume," *CanWest News Service* (May 30, 2006).

13. C. A. Slader et al., "Double Blind Randomised Controlled Trial of Two Different Breathing Techniques in the Management of Asthma," *Thorax* 61 (2006): 651–656.

14. P. Ernst et al., "Low-Dose Inhaled and Nasal Corticosteroid Use and the Risk of Cataracts," *European Respiratory Journal* 27 (2006): 1168–1174, reported in "MUHC Researchers Link Asthma Drugs And Cataracts In Seniors," *Respiratory/Asthma News* (June 4, 2006), www.medicalnewstoday.com/medicalnews.php?newsid=44500.

15. Mitchell Chavez, "Research Perspectives in Asthma: A Rationale for the Therapeutic Application of Magnesium, Pyridoxine, Coleus forskholii and Ginkgo biloba in the Treatment of Adult and Pediatric Asthma," *The Internist* 5, no. 3 (September 1998): 14–16.

Glossary

Acute. An abrupt onset, in reference to a disease. Acute often also connotes an illness that is of short duration, rapidly progressive, and in need of urgent care.

Adrenaline. A substance produced by the medulla (inside) of the adrenal gland, synonymous with epinephrine. It causes the heartbeat to quicken, strengthens the force of the heart's contraction, opens up the bronchioles in the lungs, and has numerous other effects.

Airway. The path air follows to get into and out of the lungs through the mouth and nose. Entering air then passes through the back of the throat (pharynx), continues through the voice box (larynx), down the trachea, and finally out the branching tubes known as bronchi.

Allergen. Any physical, nutritional, or emotional substance that causes an allergic response in an individual. An allergen is an antigen that usually causes an IgE (immunoglobulin E) antibody response.

Allergy. Inappropriate or exaggerated reactions of the immune system to substances that cause no symptoms in the majority of people.

Anaphylaxis. Also known as anaphylactic shock, a severe and life-threatening allergic reaction. The reaction, which is rare, can be triggered as a reaction to a drug, an insect bite, or, less commonly, after ingesting certain allergic foods.

Antigen. A substance that can trigger an immune response, resulting in the production of an antibody as part of the body's defense mechanism against allergies, infections, and disease.

Antihistamine. A drug that blocks the effects of histamine, a chemical released in body fluids during an allergic reaction.

Antioxidants. Free radical scavengers that remove dangerous free radical particles from the tissue, thereby strengthening the immune system, building up tissues, and regenerating the body.

Asthma. A chronic, inflammatory lung disease characterized by recurrent breathing problems. Asthma is often triggered by allergens, although infection, exercise, cold air, and other factors are also important triggers.

Attention deficit hyperactivity disorder. Also known as ADHD, an increasingly serious disorder common in children who lose the ability to concentrate and focus on normal daily activities. They typically become hyperactive and irritable.

Autoimmune reaction. An allergic reaction within or to one's own body or systems. Numerous autoimmune disorders exist.

B cells. Blood cells produced by the immune system to act as warriors to defend the body against invaders of any kind, including bacteria, viruses, cancer, and other medical conditions. The B cells produce antibodies or immunoglobulins.

BioSET (Bioenergetic Sensitivity and Enzyme Therapy). A natural holistic health care system that is based on energetic medicine and meridian therapy to prevent and resolve chronic health conditions. BioSET is comprised of three branches of healing: enzyme therapy to supplement nutrition and proper diet, organ-specific detoxification, and a revolutionary noninvasive, mostly permanent allergy desensitization technique.

Bronchi. Any of the larger air passages that connect the trachea (windpipe) to the lungs.

Bronchitis. An inflammation of the bronchi (lung airways), resulting in a persistent cough that produces large quantities of phlegm.

Bronchodilator drugs. A group of drugs used to expand the airways of the lungs.

Candidiasis. Also known as candida, a yeast infection that is common in asthmatics. There are numerous symptoms, including bloating, fatigue, and possible vaginal infections.

Chlorofluorocarbons (CFCs). Chemical agents that, when released into the air, can damage the earth's ozone layer. These are present in the propellants used in metered dose inhalants for asthmatics.

Chronic. Used to describe an illness that persists for a long time.

Chronic fatigue syndrome. A syndrome of multiple symptoms most commonly associated with fatigue and low energy.

Circulating immune complexes (CICs). Tiny immune complexes that float freely in the blood or the lymph fluid. They are comprised of antigens and antibodies that can be eaten by the large macrophages of the immune system.

Coenzyme Q10. Important for the production of energy in all cells of the body. It occurs naturally in the body and has been found useful in treating heart and other health problems.

Contact allergens, or contactants. Any substance that when contacted physically causes an allergic reaction. These include chemicals, fabrics, plants, and dyes.

Corticosteroids. A group of anti-inflammatory drugs commonly used to treat asthma.

Crohn's disease. An intestinal disorder associated with colitis and irritable bowel syndrome. It is an autoimmune disease.

Desensitization. A treatment to change one's reaction to an allergen or to make one less sensitive to something that is causing a reaction in the body.

Dust mites. Microscopic insect-like creatures related to the spider. They live in blankets, pillows, carpets, upholstered furniture, and curtains. Their waste products are the main components of dust, which causes many problems for asthmatics.

Eczema. An inflammation of the skin that causes itching. It is sometimes accompanied by crusting, scaling, or blisters. Many asthmatics have had or presently have eczema.

Enzymes. Complex proteins in the body that cause chemical changes in other substances in order to provide the labor force and energy necessary to keep us alive. They help convert food into chemical substances that cells can use to perform our everyday functions. They keep the immune system strong in order to fight disease and help nourish and clean the body. Life could not be sustained without enzymes.

Epinephrine. A naturally occurring hormone (also called adrenaline) released by the adrenal glands. Epinephrine dilates the airways to improve breathing and narrows blood vessels in the skin and intestine so that an increased flow of blood reaches the muscles and allows them to cope with the demands of exercise. It is the drug used to treat anaphylaxis.

Extrinsic asthma. Asthma that is triggered by an allergic reaction, usually to something that is inhaled.

Fibromyalgia. An immune complex disorder causing general fatigue and muscle aches.

Free radicals. Lone molecules that steal other molecules anywhere in the body they can find them. They are oxygen molecules that have split from their original form. In their quest for mates they cause damage to healthy tissues and cells. The results can be inflammation, cataracts, and accelerated aging.

Free-running asthma test (FRAST). A test started in 1995 to check high school students for exercise-induced asthma.

Galvanic skin response. A test involving the use of electronic devices to show any irritation to the body's electromagnetic pathways or organ systems.

Gastritis. A hyperactive condition of the stomach, also known as gastroesophageal reflux disease (GERD), that irritates the mucous membranes of the stomach, small intestines, or esophagus. It is commonly known as heartburn.

Genetic. Passing from one generation to the next. Allergies and asthma can be genetic.

Hashimoto's disease. An autoimmune disorder of the thyroid gland that causes hypothyroidism.

Hay fever. A seasonal allergy to airborne particles characterized by itchy eyes, runny nose, nasal congestion, sneezing, itchy throat, and excess mucus.

HDL. A harmful form of cholesterol.

HEPA (high-efficiency particulate arresting) filter. The most effective high-efficiency particulate air filter available for homes to remove airborne allergens harmful to asthmatics.

Histamine. A chemical present in cells throughout the body that is released during an allergic reaction. It is one of the substances responsible for the symptoms of inflammation, including sneezing and itching in allergic rhinitis. It also stimulates production of acid in the stomach and narrows the bronchi (airways) of the lungs.

Homeopathy. A natural system of medicine that uses minute doses of a remedy to cure an illness.

Homeostasis. A state of balance or equilibrium in the human body.

Hypersensitivity. An extreme sensitivity to physical, nutritional, or emotional substances that can cause symptoms in the body.

Hypoadrenal. A condition in the body where the adrenal glands are weak and do not function normally.

Hypothyroidism. A condition in the body where the thyroid gland is weak and does not function normally.

Immune system. A collection of cells and proteins that works to protect the body from potentially harmful, infectious microorganisms such as bacteria, viruses, fungi, and other disease processes.

Immunoglobulin E (IgE). An antibody that reacts with allergens to release histamines and other chemicals from cell tissues and produce allergic symptoms. When exposed to allergens, allergic individuals develop an excess of the IgE antibody.

Immunosuppressor. Anything that suppresses the immune system's ability to function normally.

Inflammation. Redness, swelling, heat, and pain in a tissue because of a chemical, physical injury, or infection. It is a characteristic of allergic reactions in the nose, lungs, and skin.

Intrinsic asthma. Asthma that has no apparent external cause.

Kinesiology. A system of healing developed by George Goodheart, DC, as a means of evaluating the human body by muscle testing and analysis. It draws upon the relationship between the muscles and organs of the body.

LDL. The good cholesterol in the body.

Lymphocytes. White blood cells of crucial importance to the adaptive part of the immune system that mounts a defense when dangerous invading organisms penetrate the body's defenses.

Mucus. A thick, slippery fluid produced by the membranes lining certain organs such as the nose, mouth, throat, and vagina. (Note that mucus is a noun while the adjective is mucous.)

Muscle response testing. A technique based on kinesiology to test a muscle, or group of muscles, in the body in relation to allergens. The BioSET system of allergy elimination uses this form of testing in its analysis.

Neurotransmitter. A biochemical substance, such as norepinephrine or acetylcholine, that transmits nerve impulses from one nerve cell to another.

Onset. In medicine, the first appearance of the signs or symptoms of an illness as, for example, the onset of rheumatoid arthritis. There is always an onset to a disease but never to the return to good health. The default setting is good health.

Pathogen. Any microorganism that can cause disease or allergies.

Peak flow monitor. An inexpensive and valuable tool for asthmatics. It measures the maximum speed with which air is forced out of the lungs and helps to monitor a worsening asthma condition. It is particularly helpful for young children who are not yet able to identify asthma symptoms.

pH. The acid-alkaline balance of the body that is so important to maintaining overall health.

Phenolics. Derivatives of benzene that are used to give flavor and color to foods and to help preserve them. There are many phenolics to which asthmatics react, and they need to be treated or desensitized to them.

Pulmonary. Having to do with the lungs.

Radioallergosorbent test (RAST). A laboratory test used to detect IgE antibodies to specific allergens.

Respiratory system. The group of organs responsible for carrying oxygen from the air to the bloodstream and for expelling the waste product, carbon dioxide.

Rotation diet. A system of treating allergies whereby a person rotates the foods they eat every few days, never eating any of the same foods more than one day in a row. It is usually a four- to five-day rotation in order to detect and eliminate food allergies.

Sick-building syndrome. Also referred to as "building-related illness." A term used when one or more occupants of a building develops similar symptoms apparently related to some indoor pollutant(s). Many of these symptoms involve hypersensitivity of the lungs and respiratory system.

Superoxide dismutase (SOD). A copper and zinc enzyme found in all body cells that is a primary defender against free radicals. SOD eliminates destructive superoxide molecules, a common free radical produced in the body, and soaks up free radical oxygen molecules in the bloodstream that would otherwise destroy healthy tissue. Some people are deficient in the enzyme and need to take it in supplemental form. SOD is found in green vegetables, yeast, sprouted seeds, and grains.

Trigger. Something that either sets off a disease in people who are genetically predisposed to developing the disease, or that causes a certain symptom to occur in a person who has a disease.

Ventilator. A machine that mechanically assists patients in the exchange of oxygen and carbon dioxide (sometimes referred to as artificial respiration).

Viral infection. An infection caused by the presence of a virus in the body. Depending on the virus and the person's state of health, various viruses can infect almost any type of body tissue, from the brain to the skin. Viral infections cannot be treated with antibiotics; in fact, in some cases the use of antibiotics makes an infection worse. The vast majority of human viral infections can be effectively fought by the body's own immune system, with a little help in the form of proper diet, hydration, and rest.

Wheezing. A whistling noise in the chest during breathing when the airways are narrowed or compressed.

Windpipe. The trachea, a tube-like portion of the respiratory (breathing) tract that connects the larynx (the voice box) with the bronchial parts of the lungs.

Bibliography

Ballentine, Rudolph. *Radical Healing*. New York: Harmony Books, 1999.

Bock, Kenneth, and Nancy Sabin. *The Road to Immunity*. New York: Pocket Books, 1998.

Crook, William G. *The Yeast Connection*. New York: Vintage Books, 1986.

Cutler, Ellen. *The Food Allergy Cure*. New York: Three Rivers Press, 2001, 2003.

Cutler, Ellen. *MicroMiracles: Discover the Healing Power of Enzymes*. New York: Rodale, 2005.

Dunne, Lavon J. *Nutrition Almanac*, 3rd ed. New York: McGraw-Hill, 1990.

Guyton, Arthur D. *Textbook of Medical Physiology*, 8th ed. Philadelphia: W. B. Saunders Company, 1991.

Hannaway, Paul J. *The Asthma Self-Help Book*. Rocklin, CA: Prima Publishing, 1992.

Jwing-Ming, Yang. *Chinese Qigong Massage*. Jamaica Plain, MA: YMAA Publication Center, 1996.

Kirschmann, Gayla J., and John D. Kirschmann. *Nutrition Almanac*, 4th ed. New York: McGraw-Hill, 1996.

Ornish, Dean. *Eat More, Weigh Less*. New York: HarperCollins Publishers, Inc., 1993.

Pennington, Jean A. T. and Anna De Planter Bowes. *Food Values*. New York: HarperCollins Publishers, 1989.

Pritikin, Robert. *The New Pritikin Program*. New York: Simon & Schuster Inc., 1990.

Saputo, Len, and Nancy Faass, eds. *Boosting Immunity*. Novato, CA: New World Library, 2002.

Vayda, William. *Attack Asthma*. Port Melbourne, Victoria: Thomas C. Lothian Pty. Ltd., 1994.

Index